Becoming a Midwife

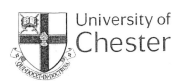

University of **Chester**

of being a midwife at the beginning of the twenty-
fi century? What is it like to help and support women throughout
pregnancy and childbirth and into motherhood. What roles can
midwives play in society?

Becoming a Midwife explores what it is to be a midwife, looking
at the factors that make midwifery such a special profession, as well
as some of the challenges. The chapters cover a variety of settings
and several different stages in a woman's pregnancy. Each one is
narrated by a midwife who introduces their own theme, recounts a
vignette that throws light on their understanding of midwifery and
reasons for becoming a midwife and any subsequent career moves.
Drawing together these insights, the editors show what it means to
be a midwife today.

Suitable for those contemplating a career in midwifery and
providing an opportunity for reflection for more experienced midwives, this thought-provoking book is an invaluable contribution
to midwifery.

Rosemary Mander is Professorial Fellow at the University of
Edinburgh, UK. She has an honorary appointment to practise as a
midwife at a local maternity unit. Her previous publications include
Caesarean and *Loss and Bereavement in Childbearing*.

Valerie Fleming is Professor of Midwifery at Glasgow Caledonian
University, UK. She is one of five mentors worldwide for the Young
Midwifery Leaders' Programme. Her previous publications includes
Failure to Progress.

Becoming a Midwife

Edited by Rosemary Mander
and Valerie Fleming

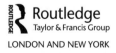

Routledge
Taylor & Francis Group

LONDON AND NEW YORK

First published 2009
by Routledge
2 Park Square, Milton Park, Abingdon, Oxon, OX14 4RN

Simultaneously published in the USA and Canada
by Routledge
270 Madison Avenue, New York, NY 10016

Reprinted 2010

Routledge is an imprint of the Taylor & Francis Group, an informa business

© 2009 Rosemary Mander and Valerie Fleming for selection and
editorial matter; individual chapters, the contributors

Typeset in Garamond by
Florence Production Ltd, Stoodleigh, Devon
Printed and bound in Great Britain by
TJ International Ltd, Padstow, Cornwall

British Library Cataloguing in Publication Data
A catalogue record for this book is available from the British Library

Library of Congress Cataloging in Publication Data
Mander, Rosemary.
  Becoming a midwife/Rosemary Mander and Valerie Fleming.
     p. cm.
  Includes bibliographical references and index.
  1. Midwifery. I. Fleming, Valerie. II. Title.
  [DNLM: 1. Midwifery. 2. Career Choice. WQ 160 M2715b 2009]
  RG950.M345 2009
  618.2 – dc22   2009008953

ISBN10: 0–415–46437–4 (hbk)
ISBN10: 0–415–46438–2 (pbk)
ISBN10: 0–203–87141–3 (ebk)

ISBN13: 978–0–415–46437–6 (hbk)
ISBN13: 978–0–415–46438–3 (pbk)
ISBN13: 978–0–203–87141–6 (ebk)

Contents

Contributors

Penny Curtis practised as a hospital-based midwife before moving to work in Central America, a move that radically changed her approach to birth. When she returned to the UK, her doctoral studies were fuelled by an interest in the ways that midwives work with, and relate to, women around birth within the bureaucratic setting of the modern hospital. Since then, Penny's interests have broadly focused on social aspects of childbearing and parenting. She also undertakes research in the area of children's health and well-being and is currently working in the School of Nursing and Midwifery at the University of Sheffield.

Jean Duerden has spent the majority of her career in midwifery, throughout which she has had a passionate respect for the supervision of midwives. This ultimately led to her appointment as an LSA Midwifery Officer for Yorkshire and Northern Lincolnshire. Prior to taking on this role, she was involved in auditing the supervision of midwives both in the north and nationally. Jean has enjoyed writing about supervision, with publications in several professional journals and chapters on supervision in eight books, including the latest edition of *Myles Textbook for Midwives*.

Allison Ewing is an Independent Midwife living in Glasgow and working all over Central Scotland. She lives only a mile away from where she grew up, but lived and worked in London for all ten years of her NHS midwifery practice. She is passionate about midwifery and revels in the reality and not just the rhetoric of 'keeping birth normal'. Allison would like to remain a clinical midwife until she retires, but this might only happen if the powers that be can find a solution to the insurance problem. She is Chair of the IM UK Database Group, supporting the Database

Coordinator. She has had two articles published in *Midwifery Matters*.

Valerie Fleming qualified as a midwife in Scotland, before working in India for a year and Thailand for six months and then settling in New Zealand. In her 16 years in New Zealand, she worked in clinical midwifery positions while completing her academic studies. Since completing her Ph.D. in 1994, Valerie has been employed as a midwife in academic institutions in New Zealand and Scotland. In addition, she has carried out consultancies in many parts of the world for the World Health Organisation (WHO) and other institutions, where her work in curriculum development is held in high esteem. She is currently Professor of Midwifery and for two years was Secretary General of the Global Network of WHO Collaborating Centres in Nursing and Midwifery.

Yvonne Fontein was born in the Netherlands where she worked in midwifery as an obstetric nurse before moving to Scotland to become a midwife. After qualification, she worked in the Netherlands as an independent midwife and continued studying at Glasgow Caledonian University. After 17 years of midwifery experience, Yvonne currently works as a lecturer and has published several midwifery-related articles.

Eleanor Forrest was born and brought up in Scotland and trained as a nurse, then midwife, in Glasgow. She has subsequently lived and worked in a variety of countries and midwifery environments over the past 27 years. Her M.Phil. was on women's experiences and perceptions of services for postnatal depression and much of her clinical experience as a midwife has focused on the care of women and families with mental health problems in the perinatal period. She was the first Glasgow-based midwife providing specialist services for perinatal mental health problems. Eleanor is currently working as a midwifery lecturer at Glasgow Caledonian University, where she has been involved in the development and delivery of modules for multiprofessional perinatal mental health practitioners. She lectures on the undergraduate midwifery programme and contributes to the internationally available postgraduate modules for midwives using a virtual learning environment.

Elaine Haycock-Stuart qualified as an adult nurse in January 1986, then became a midwife in 1988 at the General Infirmary in Leeds. After working as a staff nurse then midwife in Leeds, she moved to Edinburgh as a staff midwife and worked at the Simpson Memorial Pavilion – primarily on the postnatal ward. In 1990, she left midwifery to become a health visitor, attending Queen Margaret College with placements in the Scottish Borders. As a health visitor, Elaine worked in Forth Valley and, during her time there, studied for her doctorate at the University of Edinburgh. She became a Churchill Fellow in 1996, lectured at the University of Stirling from 1998 to 2002, and then took up her current post at the University of Edinburgh.

Ans Luyben was born, brought up and trained as a midwife and a teacher in the Netherlands. She then worked as a midwife and a teacher in institutions in the Netherlands as well as in Switzerland. Currently, she is head of a midwifery programme at the Bildungszentrum für Gesundheit und Soziales in Chur, Switzerland. Ans has carried out several small research projects and published on a variety of midwifery subjects in German, Dutch and English. Her Ph.D. addressed care during pregnancy from women's points of view in Switzerland, the Netherlands and Scotland.

Rosemary Mander practised as a midwife before moving into midwifery teaching, and then joined the University of Edinburgh. Her doctoral studies arose from her observation of poor retention of newly qualified midwives, and an interest in labour force issues continues. Her interests have moved towards the politics of maternity care, including historical and international aspects. This interest has a strong woman-centred orientation, including both the childbearing woman and the woman as a midwife. Until recently, Rosemary continued regular practice as a midwife under an honorary appointment with Lothian Health and has practised independently.

Nessa McHugh is currently a midwifery lecturer at Edinburgh Napier University and Supervisor of Midwives for Lothian Health Board. She also works as an independent midwife, carrying a caseload of her own and supporting other independent midwives. Nessa's independent practice feeds directly into her work as a lecturer, enabling her to position her teaching philosophy from the perspective of working with women in partnership. Her midwifery interests centre on feminism and the politics of childbirth.

Miranda Page feels that she wears two hats, the first as a clinical midwife working in a large and busy labour ward, the second as a researcher. Until three years ago she would have said that she was clinical first and research second. However, the tables have turned and Miranda has spent the last three years working on a Ph.D. at the Centre for Integrated Healthcare Research, where her interests lie in decision making and mother and baby attachment. If all goes well, she will complete the Ph.D. this year (2009). As to her future, maybe the tables will turn again?

Elma Paxton was born in Duns, a small town in the Scottish borders, and undertook her initial midwifery education in Stirling. Teaching qualifications were gained at Jordanhill College (now part of the University of Strathclyde) and at the University of Stirling. She has a range of cross-cultural midwifery experience, having worked in Glasgow, a very cosmopolitan city, and also through teaching and practising midwifery at the Nazareth Hospital, Israel. She is currently lecturing in midwifery at Glasgow Caledonian University, where she is Programme Leader for a well-established international B.Sc. Honours Programme in Midwifery Elma particularly enjoys deepening her understanding of midwifery in other countries and facilitating midwives towards their degrees. Her experience with pre-registration programmes also has an international dimension, as she is module leader for the student elective placement. Many students elect to travel and see practice across several continents. She is on the Board of Directors of the Edinburgh Medical Missionary Society (EMMS), which supports health projects in Malawi, India and Nepal, and maintains links with the hospital in Nazareth where she previously worked. She enjoys travel, particularly when she can combine travel with professional activities.

Lindsay Reid was born, brought up and educated in Scotland. She trained in midwifery in 1978–9 at the Royal Gwent Hospital, Newport, and has experienced midwifery from different aspects: in practice in hospital and in the community, and in education, research and writing. As Research Assistant in Midwifery, she became convinced of the need for more Scottish historical midwifery research. Her Ph.D. thesis used archival research and oral testimonies to focus on the shaping of midwives' identities in Scotland from 1916 to 1983. Lindsay's interests lie in midwifery, women's issues, writing for publication, research, both oral and archival, the need to care for and preserve archives, and history, particularly of Scotland and midwifery. She researches and writes for publication on midwifery issues and is also working on two novels based in Scotland and Shetland.

Georgina Sosa was born in 1969, at home in North London. In 1990, she started her nursing training and for one year after qualification worked in the accident and emergency department at the Royal Free Hospital in Hampstead. In 1994, she began her midwifery training at the Whittington Hospital in Archway and worked there for seven years after qualifying. She worked in all clinical areas, including the community and HM Prison, Holloway. By 2003, Georgina had married, completed a midwifery degree and M.Sc. and relocated to Norfolk. She has now worked at the James Paget University Hospitals for six years, where she practises as a clinical midwifery manager.

Denis Walsh was born and brought up in Queensland, Australia, but trained as a midwife in Leicester, UK. He has worked in a variety of midwifery environments over the past 25 years. His Ph.D. was on the Birth Centre model and he is now Associate Professor in Midwifery at the University of Nottingham. Denis lectures on evidence and skills for normal birth internationally and is widely published on midwifery issues and normal birth. He authored the best selling book, *Evidence-based Care for Normal Labour and Birth*.

Abbreviations

ARM	artificial rupture of membranes (see Glossary)
ARM	Association of Radical Midwives
CEMACH	Confidential Enquiry into Maternal and Child Health
CEMD	Confidential Enquiry into Maternal Deaths
CIS	Commonwealth of Independent States
CMB	Central Midwives Board
CTG	cardiotocograph (see Glossary)
DFID	Department for International Development
EEC	European Economic Community
EPDS	Edinburgh Postnatal Depression Scale
EU	European Union
EWTD	European Working Time Directive
FGM	female genital mutilation
FIGO	Federation International of Gynecology and Obstetrics
GP	general practitioner
HDU	high-dependency unit (see Glossary)
HE	higher education
HEI	higher education institution
IBL	inquiry-based learning
ICM	International Confederation of Midwives
IMA	Independent Midwives Association
IM-UK	Independent Midwives UK
LSA	Local Supervising Authority
LSAMO	Local Supervising Authority Midwifery Officer
ME	myalgic encephalomyelitis (see Glossary)
MSLC	Maternity Service Liaison Committee
NAS	National Archives of Scotland

NHS	National Health Service
NICE	National Institute for Health and Clinical Excellence
NIDHSS	Northern Ireland Department of Health and Social Security
NIVEL	Netherlands Institute for Health Services Research
NMC	Nursing and Midwifery Council
OP	occipito-posterior position (see Glossary)
PBL	problem-based learning
PII	professional indemnity insurance
PND	postnatal depression
PPH	post-partum haemorrhage (see Glossary)
RA	Research Assistant
RCM	Royal College of Midwives
SHHD	Scottish Home and Health Department
SHO	senior house officer
SIGN	Scottish Intercollegiate Guidelines Network
SOM	supervisor of midwives
TBA	traditional birth attendant
UK	United Kingdom
UN	United Nations
USA	United States of America
VBAC	vaginal birth after Caesarean
VSO	Voluntary Service Overseas
WHO	World Health Organisation
WHOCC	World Health Organisation Collaborating Centre
WTE	Whole Time Equivalent Midwives

Introduction

Choosing midwifery and being a midwife

Valerie Fleming and Rosemary Mander

Through the medium of this book, we are attempting to explore the nature and meaning of midwifery. Our intention is that this exploration will help two possibly rather different groups of people who are contemplating midwifery. On the one hand, you may be contemplating midwifery because you are considering entering it with a view to making a career as a midwife; this may be either as a first career or as a career change later in life. On the other hand, you may be an experienced and highly expert midwife who is taking an opportunity to reflect on your future career. This book is intended to provide food for thought that will help you with making these crucially important decisions.

Midwifery as a practice discipline

This book aims to explore midwifery from a number of different viewpoints. These different perspectives matter. This is because the midwife's point of view tends to be neglected due to, unsurprisingly, the midwife's main focus being on those for whom she provides care. Thus, less is written about the way in which the midwife views midwifery in general and her own job in particular. A factor that is consistent throughout midwifery, though, is the fundamental nature of midwifery as a form of practice. While there may be any number of ways of approaching, analysing or explaining midwifery, they all come down to the primacy of the actual activities or behaviour of the midwife, which become evident in the process of attending a childbearing woman. In spite of all the technological developments in maternity care, it is the practice of the midwife that continues to provide the essential focus for all those involved in midwifery. The essential nature of practice is clearly apparent in the International Confederation of Midwives (ICM) (WHO/ICM/ FIGO 2005) definition, which we quote later in this introductory chapter.

Having recognised the centrality of practice and the crucial place of the midwife's relationship with the childbearing woman, it may now be helpful to broaden the area of scrutiny. This broader view is necessary in order to access the variety of midwifery-based activities that serve to support and, possibly, enhance the role of the practitioner. This range of activities is probably infinite, but it includes the educator, the supervisor and the manager, to name but three.

Although the focus and centrality of midwifery practice are unalterable, as we have argued already, that practice and those related activities are certainly not. This is in part because of the technological changes in health care, and in part because of the increasing evidence base, which serves to facilitate ever more effective midwifery practice. Additionally, there is a multitude of other developments that impinge on the midwife and her client. Because of these constantly changing influences, we should regard the midwifery profession as a dynamic system that is constantly adjusting and readjusting to a multiplicity of developments. While some of these adjustments are reactive in response to changes in, for example, consumer demands, a large proportion of them will be proactive through the development of new ideas and research.

Perceptions of the midwife's role

The chapters in this book will help us to consider how the midwife's role is perceived, in terms of the various roles that the midwife may assume. This perspective will introduce the changes in and about midwifery that impinge on the midwife's functioning. In order to do this, the midwife's various roles are scrutinised, together with reflections on their relationship with midwifery theory and with midwifery practice.

As we discuss in the Conclusion, perceptions about what the midwife actually does may be in need of the attention that this book offers. One group who may need particular help in achieving this understanding is among those who are likely to be reading this book. There continues to be a small number of people who, trained as nurses, become interested in a career in midwifery. It may be that these 'converts' are the nurses who are best placed to understand the differences between nursing and midwifery.

For some, though, such understanding may present difficulties. Such difficulties may be, in part, due to the organisation of the health professions, through the introduction of statutory bodies such as the Nursing and Midwifery Council (NMC). While the relationship between nurses and midwives is generally harmonious and constructive, there are occasional rumblings, which may suggest that a small number see the situation differently (Thompson *et al.* 2007). Such misconceptions will, hopefully, be corrected through the medium of this book. As mentioned already, midwives' forte may not necessarily be found in their accounts of the underpinnings of their own practice. So such misconceptions may not be unique to these authors; in fact they may not be alone in their limited understanding of what midwives actually do to support women and ensure healthy outcomes for those in their care.

Therefore, this book, as well as providing information for potential and experienced midwives, will assist in dispelling the misconceptions and incorrect assumptions made by a wide range of interested parties. While some of the perceptions may be of what some might call the more mundane aspects of midwifery, these will be supported and enhanced by the profound nature of the accompanying reflections. This deeper, more reflective level will show the intense significance that the midwife attaches to the midwifery role. As may be helpful with any truly profound abstract reflection, stories in the form of vignettes will be used to illustrate its significance. While a picture has been said to 'speak a thousand words', we would like to suggest that a good story speaks volumes.

Contemplating midwifery

By way of an introduction to midwifery and to assist both groups for whom this book is intended, it is helpful to contemplate the reasons for embarking on a career in midwifery. This contemplation will resonate particularly for you if you are considering entering midwifery. Additionally, though, this contemplation will serve to remind the more experienced midwife of her reasons for becoming a midwife.

People choosing to become midwives do so for many different reasons. Most are enthusiastic about helping women through pregnancy, to give birth or in the postnatal period. Some people who become midwifery students will have come straight from school.

Many others, though, will choose midwifery as a second career, perhaps having had experience of childbirth. Others still will be graduates from other disciplines who decide upon a different career. Current students, reflecting each of these cohorts, tell of some of their own reasons for choosing the profession.

Hannah's story

Like many other young people in the UK today, my education has been an extensive one. Soon to graduate from my second degree, it is an apt time to reflect on the choices I have made and the lessons I have learnt. Leaving secondary school I knew I was interested in two divergent subjects, the creative arts and midwifery. Two very different career paths, yet both reflective of my personality. At the age of 19 I was accepted into the Glasgow School of Art to study textiles, which began as a very exciting and self-defining opportunity. Throughout the next four years I [gained] a great appreciation of the tactile qualities that textiles offer. However, the learning process, I found, was individually focused [and] competitive and I was therefore subject to criticism . . . not always constructive. Once graduated I was thrown into the cut-throat world [in which] all designers find themselves. Fighting for positions and exploited in terms of both time and money. After some time I realised that this career path was not fulfilling and my attention turned to my other interest – midwifery.

Entering the course I was instantly surprised by the difference in the teaching process and collaborative nature of the course. Participating in group projects and inquiry-based learning, combined with supportive tutors (who are always constructive!), I found that I thrived. However, I did find that my previous expertise in textiles was not to be dismissed; the once divergent paths did in fact [run] parallel. During my second-year group presentation (a project entailing presenting and disseminating information on the topic of domestic abuse to peers), I discovered I was able to communicate my ideas through images and text. I also contributed to a small project called 'The Mum's Make It Project', which encouraged young teenage mothers to use art and being creative as a therapeutic and social tool. Through this project and utilising both my creative and midwifery skills I felt I had discovered a way to truly be 'with women', which, in turn, finally gave me a sense of fulfilment and contentment.

(Hannah Wright 2008)

Christine's story

I left school at 15 with no idea what I wanted to do. I found out that a local college offered a direct access course which ran in conjunction with the university. This was great for me; if I passed all my modules at college I was guaranteed admission to university, which was something I never thought that I would be able to do. I am now incredibly grateful that this option was there for me as I now love what I am doing, though the studying is tough with kids and placements and essays, but it is do-able!

(Christine Craig 2008)

Laura's story

Prior to my application to midwifery, I arranged, myself, to spend a week's work experience at a maternity unit. Considering I was planning on starting university straight after leaving school, I thought this was extremely valuable in giving me a realistic view of my future career. I learnt a lot about the different aspects of maternity care, from conception through to the handover to the health visitor. I would recommend that anyone planning on applying for a midwifery course gets some form of work experience, so that you know what the job entails.

(Laura Meiklejohn 2008)

Heather's story

When I told my family that I wanted to become a midwife, they were a little bit surprised! I already have a degree in art history, and for the three years after finishing my degree I had worked in retail management, so this was a slight deviation from what I had been doing. However, it was one of the shops that I worked in that started to give me the idea of what I wanted to do with my life. I worked for two years as the manager of a maternity wear shop, and I realised after talking to all the women that I dealt with that I found the whole process of pregnancy and midwifery really interesting, so I then started to look into midwifery and what I would need to gain access to the course. My sister at the same time was also pregnant, so I was able to see what care my sister received and a better idea if midwifery was something I could do and enjoy. So I then went on to do some researching online, looking at different universities and courses. I emailed Catriona (the admissions tutor) and asked her about entry qualifications, and she said that I would need an updated science qualification because my degree was arts based. So I got a job and started night school to complete my higher in Human Biology! I then had to wait and see if I would get an interview, so it was a scary process! I was doing a higher that I might not have needed; luckily I like biology so I didn't mind!

I got the interview!! I was so excited but at the same time oh so very nervous!! I was interviewed by Catriona and another senior midwife from one of the units, and I remember just telling myself to be me because that's the person who would have to be a midwife so no point trying to be someone false. I left the interview thinking that it went well, but it was hard to tell. So it was back to work to wait and see if I would get a place in the course! Scary!!

I was on holiday in Malaysia when my sister phoned me saying that my letter had arrived .... eek!! So she opened it and told me that I had my place, on the condition that I got a C or above in my higher! I started crying and it was a very happy moment!! Luckily I got a B for my higher and in September 2006 I started the journey to become a midwife!

(Heather Burt 2008)

Tomoko's story

I decided to do midwifery when I had my first child 10 years ago. I thought about it for a while and started to look into midwifery courses. I didn't meet entry requirements at the time – my qualifications from a different country were not recognised. When my daughter turned one, I started college and gained some general qualifications. In addition, I got interested in aromatherapy so gained a diploma in aromatherapy followed by a teaching certificate in baby massage. I hoped that when I qualify as a midwife I could incorporate these skills in my care.

I also looked for a job in hospital/care setting to gain some experience. I knew some care experience was desirable in applicants so I took a job as a phlebotomist, which I still do several years on. In addition to these, I went to see the admissions tutor at the university and discussed what else I could do to help me get into midwifery. I did my own research into midwifery and spoke to some of my midwife friends to find out more.

Luckily, I did get into midwifery straight away and took the first step in my dream career. To be honest, I was not very confident in my academic ability, but I put effort into my work and I somehow managed to sail through to the final year. Clinical placements are very important and I feel I learned most of my midwifery skills on placement. Lectures are good to attend, but I would say I obtained information mainly from doing literature searches/reading books in my own time. The lecturers are all nice and they are always there if I need help.

(Tomoko Pearl 2008)

Regardless of their reason for choosing midwifery, it is important that both potential and experienced midwives keep in mind the international definition of the midwife:

A midwife is a person who, having been regularly admitted to a midwifery educational programme, duly recognised in the country in which it is located, has successfully completed the prescribed course of studies in midwifery and has acquired the requisite qualifications to be registered and/or legally licensed to practise midwifery.

The midwife is recognised as a responsible and accountable professional who works in partnership with women to give the necessary support, care and advice during pregnancy, labour and the postpartum period, to conduct births on the midwife's own responsibility and to provide care for the newborn and the infant. This care includes preventative measures, the promotion of normal birth, the detection of complications in mother and child, the accessing of medical care or other appropriate assistance and the carrying out of emergency measures.

The midwife has an important task in health counselling and education, not only for the woman, but also within the family and the community. This work should involve antenatal education and preparation for parenthood and may extend to women's health, sexual or reproductive health and child care.

A midwife may practise in any setting including the home, community, hospitals, clinics or health units.

(WHO/ICM/FIGO 2005)

Being students

Midwifery students, like midwives, thus come from many backgrounds and are a variety of ages. As with any other students, all of them have highs and lows throughout their educational programme. However, from the beginning, because classes are generally small, strong bonds are formed and it is often during these lows that the support of classmates can help.

Skills students bring to the programme can also make a valuable contribution to existing projects. This was particularly the case for one group of students who made a group presentation on Domestic Abuse (see Figure I.1).

These presentations and other forms of learning prepare students to become midwives, but what of the world of midwifery?

This book outlines many career pathways available for midwives. Some of these may be new, but both potential and experienced midwives are advised to think about these and others so that they can tailor their education programme towards a final goal. While most of the chapters in this book discuss midwifery careers in the United Kingdom (UK), we must remember that we have a lot to learn from midwifery elsewhere. For this reason, some chapters have been included to stimulate thoughts on midwifery as a global profession, keeping in mind that the midwife of today may work in several countries. In selecting their midwifery education, prospective students and experienced midwives should consider the choices available in light of future aspirations.

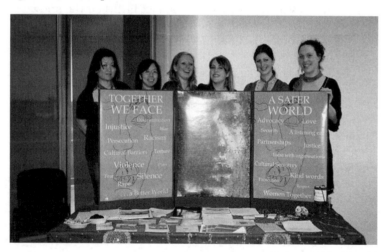

Figure I.1 Student presentation: from left to right, Tomoko Pearl, Hau-Yin Tsang, Claire Sheridan, Hannah Wright, Kathryn Openshaw and Rhona Shrestha.
Source: Photo courtesy of Gillian Lang, midwifery tutor and project facilitator (2008).

The arrangement of the chapters in this book

Through the use of real-life vignettes, each chapter will focus on a different aspect of midwifery to indicate the factors that generate dynamism within the profession. These dynamics will emerge through the midwife's reflection on the experience-based vignette that she or he has chosen to recount. This vignette-oriented reflection will be related to what it was that brought the midwife to enter midwifery in the first place, which may or may not be the same as what keeps the midwife in midwifery. Through these reflections, what will manifest itself is the meaning of midwifery to the midwives who practice it. The commentaries, summaries and reflections of the editors will serve to draw out the linkages and themes that happen to unite the chapters by the very different individuals who are the midwife contributors.

In this way, the first purpose of this book is to highlight, for the potential or new midwife, the opportunities that are likely to present themselves. Also provided will be much food for thought, which the potential or new midwife may need to consider before embarking on this new career. As well as providing a guide for the new midwife, this book will also offer an opportunity for the more experienced and expert midwife to undertake a 'reality check'. This will facilitate reflection on the position of the expert midwife and of midwifery in the wider health care system and in the world as a whole. Such reflection is likely to assist practitioners and others in making decisions about their future career development.

The first part of the book concentrates on those aspects of the midwifery role that come most easily to mind. These are the characteristics of midwifery that relate to working with women in an institution, such as a National Health Service (NHS) hospital. In order to emphasise the centrality of the woman to midwifery practice, the first part will be organised according to the childbearing woman's experience of maternity and midwifery care.

The second part of the book looks at aspects of midwifery that are not so widely known. These aspects will be addressed in order to demonstrate the career opportunities for those entering midwifery. This material is also likely to be valuable to more experienced midwives contemplating their careers. There will also be an attempt to address the issues raised by these roles. In order to broaden the readers' horizons, the international orientation will be more pronounced in the second part.

References

Thompson, D.R., Watson, R. and Stewart, S. (2007) 'Guest editorial – Nursing and midwifery: time for an amicable divorce?', *International Journal of Nursing Studies* 44(4): 523–4.

World Health Organisation/International Confederation of Midwives/ International Federation of Gynecology and Obstetrics (WHO/ICM/ FIGO) (2005) *Definition of the Midwife*, Geneva: WHO.

Part 1

The midwife and the institution

Chapter 1

Midwifery care in the community during the woman's pregnancy

Yvonne Fontein

'Pregnant, but not happy', that's how I felt. After all these years I was finally pregnant but I did not feel happy and I was scared to tell anyone. That was until today, when meeting my midwife changed my feelings somehow. I was very apprehensive to go and see her and did not plan to share my feelings with her. But somehow she managed to ask all the right questions, to recognise my worries and to give me the feeling that I am actually allowed to feel this. When she and I listened to the baby's heartbeat it made me realise there is really a baby growing in me. Although I am glad we still have a long way to go before this baby will arrive, somehow I think I will be able to get through this and to start enjoying what is ahead of me, and I am sure there is someone out there to look after me and this baby.

Stories such as this made me realise that pregnancy is a major event in the life of a woman and her family and represents a journey to motherhood. How to become a caring, safe and considerate midwife to accompany the woman's journey is influenced by the fact that every woman is unique, each pregnancy is an original journey and every experience is special. There appears to be no such thing as an average woman in an ordinary community needing routine care. This kindled my interest in becoming a midwife.

The woman's pregnancy and the midwife

There are ideas and philosophies that form the foundations of how the midwife takes care of a woman during her pregnancy – known as antenatal care. Although midwives have been doing this for centuries, these ideas are given such names as *holistic midwifery, woman-centred care, partnership, assessment of well-being* and *multidisciplinary care*. These ideas and philosophies need some explanation to understand them and how a midwife can use them to underpin her work while caring for pregnant women, and how they are incorporated and experienced by the midwife on a day-to-day basis.

Holistic midwifery

Pregnancy is represented by the physical changes in the woman's body. However, it also involves other dimensions of the woman, such as her mind or emotions. One aspect can influence the other; if a woman is feeling very unhappy, this can have an effect on her physical condition in pregnancy, as anxieties and worries can cause an imbalance in a pregnant woman's physical health. The woman's relationship with her partner, family circumstances, housing, worries about motherhood, work and finances are examples that can influence to women's health and can, for example, affect blood pressure or cause morning sickness. A woman can experience feelings of guilt towards her unborn baby when she smokes, or her altering body image, as a result of pregnancy, can make a woman feel unattractive and cause feelings of depression. As these are very normal day-to-day aspects of pregnancy, this illustrates that pregnancy is not a just a physical experience that can be separated from the woman as a whole.

To address the full context of the woman and her pregnancy as a total integrated concept is called *holistic midwifery* (Walsh and Steen 2007). Taking into account the whole concept of the woman's emotional, psychological, social, physical, cultural, spiritual needs and expectations and their relationship makes a midwife a *holistic midwife*.

Woman-centred care

Pregnancy is an experience in a woman's life that has a different value or meaning to every individual woman. When a woman presents herself for her first antenatal visit, the midwife has to appreciate that a woman brings in her experiences of the past, her present needs and her expectations and hopes for the future. Although it is the element and presence of pregnancy itself that brings the woman into contact with the midwife, the woman also brings with her this total package of herself, her being and the community she is part of. Recognising, acknowledging and respecting the individual woman and her unique needs, ideas, thoughts, emotions, expectations and wishes about pregnancy, motherhood and childbirth related issues, is known as *woman-centred care*, in other words: the woman and her unborn baby come first (Leap and Homer 2002).

Partnership

The concept of working in *partnership* with a woman is an important contributing factor for the midwife to achieve woman-centered care. This means a process of teamwork between a woman, her partner or significant others and the midwife, working towards a shared goal, which can entail all sorts of issues such as place of birth and so on – in general, a healthy pregnancy and a healthy baby. Partnership is characterised by an exchange of the midwife's knowledge and expertise and the woman's expectations, needs, anxieties and experiences. The midwife contributes her or his knowledge and professional experience and the woman brings her package of personal needs, wishes, questions, uncertainties or anxieties. The midwife has to give sound information to a woman to offer her realistic choices in relation to topics such as antenatal tests, but also to make her aware of the choices available. Therefore, it is an exchange of information between the midwife and the woman; the midwife has the responsibility to inform a woman about her options and choices, while the woman has to inform the midwife of her needs in order to address them. This implies that both the woman and the midwife contribute to the relationship they have, which is focused on the pregnancy and the journey into motherhood. The fact that both the woman and the midwife are contributing to the childbirth experience from a different angle and background enhances the professional role and responsibility of the midwife as well as the personal part the woman plays in this joint adventure of childbirth.

Assessment of well-being

Pregnancy and antenatal care are not independent or isolated parts of midwifery care, but are integral parts of the whole childbirth process. Assessment of well-being is known to be effective in measuring the woman's and baby's health, but also in detecting if well-being is threatened. To assess well-being the midwife has to have practical skills, such as recording blood pressure, measuring the growth of the foetus, listening to the foetal heartbeat, taking bloods, estimating the date of the baby's birth or administering medication. In the definition of the midwife (see page 7 in the Introduction) it is acknowledged that the midwife is responsible for detecting complications in mother and child. In order to ensure this happens, the midwife has to have substantial knowledge of the woman's anatomy, how the body works and what happens and changes during pregnancy, as well as skills to examine this. The midwife has in-depth knowledge of the normal progression of pregnancy, the bodily and psychological changes and the common discomforts and is able to understand the normal results of basic screening laboratory tests, such as iron levels and urine testing.

When caring for pregnant women, the midwife has a breadth of knowledge and a wealth of expertise. The midwife does not regard pregnancy as an illness, but as a normal life event, and has confidence in and trusts and respects the childbirth process and the woman's capabilities in childbirth (ICM 2005). The midwife's extensive knowledge and insight into the woman's body and pregnancy are necessary to establish if a pregnant woman and her baby are progressing and developing, as can be expected in a healthy situation. *Normal*, *healthy* and *physiological* are all terms to describe the midwife's professional domain and responsibility. Only women fulfilling these requirements of *normality* can be cared for by the midwife. This does not mean that the midwife has no knowledge of what is abnormal, unhealthy or pathological, but that this does not belong to the midwife's professional sphere of practice. The midwife is, however, very much aware of possible adverse effects on the health and well-being of a woman and her baby if complications arise. At the moment that the midwife detects an abnormal situation or complication in the pregnancy, the she or he is no longer able to give adequate and responsible care and will therefore access appropriate medical care (ICM 2005). Every aspect of the woman's pregnancy that is examined, discovered and discussed needs to be documented. Sometimes, women have their own personal notes and take these wherever they go, whatever happens or whomever they see in pregnancy.

Multidisciplinary care

The midwife works collaboratively with other health care professionals, such as general practitioners, obstetricians, paediatricians, health visitors and physiotherapists. The midwife will consult or refer to an appropriate health professional if she or he detects any signs of complications during the woman's pregnancy needing further examination outside the midwife's knowledge and responsibility (ICM 2002). Therefore, the midwife's documentation of the woman's pregnancy is an important tool to assist in the procedure of consultation or referral and to make sure that all the health professionals involved know what the midwife has observed and done.

Situations can arise in which a woman's pregnancy has to be monitored and cared for in the hospital under the supervision of an obstetrician, whose professional domain includes, unlike the midwife, complications in childbirth. Although pregnancy is a healthy event, it sometimes deteriorates into an unhealthy or dangerous situation for mother and baby. In such cases, the midwife is no longer allowed to be the woman's primary care provider. The woman may be admitted to hospital to be cared for, or stay at home and go to the hospital to be examined. The midwife may visit the woman in the hospital or at home to share her experiences and to support her, although the duty of care is handed over to the obstetrician. Whatever complications have arisen, it is hoped that they will disappear and the woman can go home, where care will be taken over again by the midwife.

Reflection

Midwifery can be regarded as a maturing profession, especially for young midwives. During antenatal visits, a woman sometimes shares very private, intimate and confidential information with the midwife about what is going on in her life. These can be aspects of life that sometimes have a shocking element. On the one hand, it is a privilege to be confided in by the woman – her personal thoughts, emotions and life circumstances; on the other hand, being confided in needs to be dealt with in a cautious and professional way.

When a woman presents herself for the first time during pregnancy, she may share her history with the midwife. A woman's story may very well include abortion, homosexual relationships, sexually transmitted diseases, drug abuse, domestic abuse or other very personal issues with a highly moral, ethically significant or social stigma. The midwife also probably has personal thoughts, ideas or even experiences in regard to these issues. Sometimes, it is difficult for a woman to give this information, especially at a first acquaintance, but for the midwife it can also be very challenging and demanding not to give a personal opinion. When a midwife is being confronted with difficult life issues or ethical dilemmas, at any stage of the midwife's professional development or career, it is important to reflect on his or her own ideas, values, beliefs, thoughts and feelings, and how to prevent these from influencing the midwife's care for or communication with the woman.

Midwifery is often regarded as a 'happy profession', as it involves the happy events of pregnancy and birth and, fortunately, this is often very true. However, despite all our knowledge and medical support, sadly a pregnancy occasionally does not have a good or happy outcome and can compromise the woman's or unborn baby's health, sometimes resulting in death. Although life and death are both events belonging to life, it can be very hard to accept that death can belong to pregnancy. In difficult situations, the midwife has not only to cope with the woman's and her partner's feelings, but also with personal emotions. It is very important to be aware of personal feelings in relation to sensitive and emotionally complex situations, as well as to be able to put these aside as subordinate to the woman's opinions and emotions. It therefore needs not only professional and personal growth and development, but also a high level of self-awareness and reflection from the midwife to be non-judgemental, to show that you care, sometimes to shed a tear, but also to keep a professional distance, and that all at the same time. For midwifery students or young midwives it can be difficult when they seek out their friends or peers to share their experiences with or to look for comfort or a shoulder to cry on. Friends may have chosen other professions or career paths and may find it hard to understand what midwifery encompasses. Fortunately, midwives are not alone but are surrounded by other midwives and health professionals to share experiences and emotions with.

The journey

At the moment a woman finds out that she is pregnant, she envisages her future and what this will be like in nine months' time. The journey of pregnancy and preparation for motherhood starts at the very beginning of the pregnancy, when a woman attends her first antenatal visit; a midwife is privileged to make the journey of childbirth with a woman and her significant others, to support them, facilitate them in the process and guide them through their journey. However, the period of pregnancy is time-restricted, as it lasts for approximately 40 weeks. Pregnancy is, therefore, a short but intense period leading into motherhood, which in itself is a lifelong event and will eventually integrate into a woman's life as it continues on its path. Although the midwife only participates in a short episode in the woman's journey through life on the whole, it is obvious that he or she has an important role to play in the short but profound time-span of pregnancy and birth. The midwife accompanies the woman and her family, starting at the beginning of pregnancy, aiming to prepare and equip them as best as can be achieved for the journey ahead. This is not a routine job because it impacts on the individual life of a woman, her partner and family, regardless of the outcome of the pregnancy. Every year a child's birthday is going to be celebrated; what the midwife said or did at the time is going to be recalled. An experienced midwife describes it:

If the voyage of childbirth can be seen as a metaphor of a train journey; the midwife embarks the train in pregnancy and disembarks shortly after the birth of the baby, waves them good-bye and wishes them a further safe and pleasant journey.

Although a midwife is predominantly involved in a one-to-one situation with a woman, this is not entirely true, as a woman is part of a family, a social network and a community.

Midwifery care in the community

A midwife may practise in any setting, including the community and the woman's home (ICM 2005). Although the woman comes first and is the centre of the midwife's care, she cannot be separated from the community she lives in. Historically, the midwife always had, and still has, a position and place in the community, serving the childbearing population in a specific area. In the community the midwife can be based in a health centre or a general practitioner's surgery, but the working environment can also include the woman's home.

Midwives work among various populations, each with their specific characteristics, such as level of education or affluence, religion or origin, as well as local health problems and needs or special needs in relation to childbirth. Midwives may be practising within the same country, area or even in the same town, but their care can comprise and focus on completely different aspects. A midwife can be located in a poor area with mixed cultures, including minority groups, where single motherhood, teenage pregnancy and substance abuse frequently occur and where women's own mothers or peers are their informants. Midwifery care here will differ from that of a midwife in an affluent area, with older first-time mothers in stable relationships with established careers, who maybe had to seek medical assistance to become pregnant and who use the internet as their primary source of information. Differences in midwifery care can also be affected and influenced by the level of urbanisation of the community in which the midwife is positioned. The midwife can be based in a city or town where women live near to hospitals and can access maternity services easily. The midwife can also work rurally, where the infrastructure differs from that of an urban area, where women live at a distance from maternity facilities, where pregnancy is a widely accepted aspect of life not needing a lot of fuss or specific attention, and where home birth is the norm. A woman has to be recognised within the wider picture of the society in which she lives, as this influences the woman's perception and experience of the pregnancy and her preparation for motherhood. This needs to be a key aim for the midwife.

Significant others

The minute a woman discovers that she is pregnant, she instantly thinks how this is going to affect her current life, her family, her work, study or benefits and her social life. Whether it is a first baby or a subsequent child, a planned or unplanned pregnancy, life will be deeply affected by expecting a baby and everything that this possibly may imply for the future. The news of a pregnancy can bring joy but also worries, and can be accepted unconditionally or with reservation, depending on personal and living circumstances.

A pregnancy will change the woman into a mother, her partner into a father, other children into brothers or sisters and parents into grandparents. All these individuals will react and respond to the pregnancy in their own way as it has different effects, meanings or values for each of them. If a woman is the first to become pregnant among her friends, she may lose some of those friends as a result of entering a phase in her life not understood by peers. It may, however, enhance or bring about friendships with others who already have children. Maybe there are friends or family members who would like to have children but who have not yet succeeded in getting pregnant or who have had a miscarriage; a woman may be very apprehensive in approaching them to give them the news of her pregnancy, not wanting to hurt them. All these people, those who are important and near to the woman, are known as her *significant others*. How these significant others respond to the pregnancy can affect how the woman experiences her pregnancy, either positively or negatively. Employers can also influence how the woman undergoes her pregnancy, especially in relation to the contents of her work and how or if this integrates with a pregnancy, as well as the consideration of whether the woman wants to return to work after her pregnancy.

For the midwife, these are important aspects to be aware of in order not only to assess how these possibly influence the woman's pregnancy and her process into motherhood, but also to put the woman in the context of her social background. Issues to be discussed during the antenatal period are the woman's home situation, for example does she live with her partner or at home with her parents, is the pregnancy planned and wanted, does she have a job and, if so, can it be combined with her pregnancy? Is the woman going to return to work, is she financial independent or are there other sources to provide for the baby and is there is a social network that supports the woman? Discussing personal issues such as these requires huge interest and involvement from the midwife and a trusting relationship with the woman. Sometimes, close involvement with a woman and her significant others means that the midwife suspects or becomes aware of difficult situations, such as domestic violence. Fortunately, the midwife can share these problems with the woman's general practitioner (GP) or health visitor, who are also involved in the woman's health and that of her family. To understand how the social network of significant others is structured gives the midwife insight into the woman's home situation and her community of family and friends. Regardless of the outcome of the pregnancy, even if a pregnancy results in a miscarriage, it is this small community the midwife would try to involve in order to support the woman in her home environment. A part-time midwife describes her involvement:

I always know what is going on with my women and in their families and how they are all related, who had a baby or lost it, who had a miscarriage, who get on and who don't, who is ill or who died; even when I am not working. It sounds like gossiping but it isn't, I am interested in my women and their families. When I am doing my antenatal visits sometimes women do not have to say anything because I know. It makes me feel part of it all, I belong and stand next to them as being part of their community, their life . . . My friend who works in [town] has a huge caseload, much bigger than mine and she says it is difficult with so many women and all different cultures to build a good relationship with her women. I suppose it is not everybody's cup of tea anyway . . . .

Working in the woman's home and the health centre

Antenatal care takes place in the health centre as well as in the woman's home, depending on the woman's wishes or circumstances. Circumstances can dictate that a woman may not be able to keep her antenatal appointments, for reasons unknown to the midwife. Inviting or letting the midwife into the home means that the woman does not have to travel to the midwife or have to wait for lengths of time in a surgery's waiting room, which could be full of sick people. It also means, however, being vulnerable when there are visible problems to be observed, such as poverty. Being in the woman's home means that the midwife is the guest and the woman is in control in her environment, while in the health centre, being the midwife's territory, it is the midwife who is in control. In contrast to a clinical health centre or surgery, the personal and individual atmosphere of the woman's home gives the midwife an impression about her home environment and family life, which would have otherwise remained unknown. When a woman is considering a home birth, practicalities are best discussed in the woman's home, where the midwife can assess possibilities for or hindrances to this event. Two midwives describe their experiences:

Sometimes you have this image of a woman; how she lives, her partner, etc. Then you visit her at her house and this image can just shatter to pieces as it is so different than you expected. For me it can put a woman into a wider perspective, picture her better, and I sometimes find it easier to understand a woman, having seen what she is talking about.

I love to do antenatal home visits, it makes it so much more personal . . . I mean most women are so much more relaxed. If I am busy though, the health centre is so much more convenient; all my equipment is there and I just refer women to the reception for their next appointment. You have to watch the clock though because somebody else will be waiting, so if you want to discuss things properly, there is hardly any time and you're always feeling the pressure that you have to hurry.

Local community

Women come from a variety of social backgrounds, ages, religions, family settings or political status, such as asylum seekers or refugees. Perceptions of pregnancy and preparation for motherhood are related to their backgrounds and to personal experiences with pregnancy or motherhood. Ideas, thoughts and fears of childbirth are embedded in a woman's personal circumstances as well as in the wider context of the society she lives in.

When a midwife works in a local community she is familiar with the population in her area, such as levels of affluence and employment, size of local population, housing, cultural diversity, religion, infrastructure such as the accessibility of shops, childcare, health care and emergency services. Statistics in the area of home births and breastfeeding, existing social problems or health issues, for example smoking or teenage pregnancies, are known to the midwife. These facts and figures affect the childbearing population and therefore form the contents of the midwife's parenthood education, which is an important task in antenatal care. The midwife often deals with these issues on an individual level, but also provides this valuable information to groups in the woman's community. On an individual level, the woman can discuss a *birth plan* with the midwife, which is a written plan where the woman records her personal ideas and wishes about the forthcoming birth, for example positioning during birth, the role of her partner or skin-to-skin contact with the baby.

Parenthood education

Groups for parenthood education consist of pregnant women from the community and focus on explanation of the birth process, techniques for relaxation, coping with childbirth, choices in place of birth and method of feeding (ICM 2002). As well as the fact that relevant information is provided, these groups give women a chance for social interaction and often these remain in place after babies are born, sometimes resulting in long-term friendships. This provides the opportunity for women to share their experiences and the practicalities of pregnancy and later to share their birth stories or their experiences with a newborn baby. The midwife facilitates breastfeeding support groups not only for mothers, but also for pregnant women interested in breastfeeding. In these groups the midwife gives relevant information, stimulates the sharing of information among women and also learns from women's experiences, adding this to his or her own professional knowledge and expertise. Because of the mixed nature of the groups, with both first-time and experienced mothers, women can exchange their experiences, their anxieties and hopes and can learn from each other. Women will meet each other again at the health visitor's, playgroup, nursery and later at the local school. It is a nice aspect of the midwife's job to see friendships flourish during the antenatal period, knowing that an aspect of midwifery is to facilitate the exchange of personal experiences and the development of relationships. Partners or other significant others are often invited to join women during parenthood education sessions, not only to learn and share information, but also to feel acknowledged in a supporting role.

Midwives often refer to women in the community as *their women*, which illustrates the involvement and personal aspect of the relationship between the woman and the midwife, which can have advantages and disadvantages. One midwife describes the advantages:

After living and working in the same area for all these years, it is lovely to see these mums and their children in the streets, knowing I have been involved with all of them and to see them grow up and to remember anecdotes from when they were pregnant.

Another midwife says:

There are times that it is impossible to 'just pop into the shops' to get my last minute shopping, as I bump into all these mothers with prams wanting to show their baby, share their stories or ask questions about nappy rash or breastfeeding. This is one of the reasons that my own daughter never wants to come to the shops with me as 'I am always talking to everyone'.

Day-to-day practice

The midwife's work is a fusion of knowledge and competencies and it is a composite of a variety of skills that are incorporated into day-to-day practice. Practical skills, such as record keeping, are utilised during antenatal visits alongside a range of counselling and communication skills, all performed with a professional attitude and knowledge. On the one hand, assessing well-being is the main focus of antenatal care, but, on the other hand, antenatal care comprises immense variety and diversity. All skills are applied in a day's work during which the midwife meets pregnant women, assesses their pregnancies and well-being, provides the necessary information, listens to their worries and thoughts, tries to address their needs, supports them in making choices, documents findings, makes appointments for future visits, refers women to other appropriate health professionals and provides education. All of these issues are addressed when a single antenatal visit is often restricted to ten minutes. Antenatal care is dynamic and the midwife will hardly experience a dull moment when involved with women and their families.

First-year midwifery students describe their thoughts about antenatal care and how women can perceive this:

I think the thing that I am finding the most inspiring about the antenatal care is the foetal heartbeat. The other examinations, urine, blood and explanations for why we are doing them is really interesting after university study and because it offers a complete picture, etc. but I hadn't considered the impact of those first aural moments especially for the new mums (obviously some are completely unmoved and carry on chewing their gum!); but on the whole that second when the heartbeat beeps in on the machine and you turn it up and it's galloping away is just brilliant – I suppose I will become quite accustomed to this when I have heard a lot of them but at the moment it is wonderful every time and even someone who would never want to be a midwife would find this absolutely amazing – I did one [heartbeat] today with both mum and granny in the room and all three of us were in tears (very unprofessional I'm sure).

Another student describes the emotional involvement and the awareness of professional distance, but also the diversity of the midwife's role, in that it does not only involve supporting women giving birth and smiling happy faces:

A lot of the girls going out on placement have been talking about the emotional side of midwifery . . . some weren't sure whether it was ok to

have a wee cry along with the mother at something beautiful, sad etc.
... I wasn't sure, but, apparently (according to one of the mentors), it's
the only health profession you get to show any emotion in, and get away
with it. Another comment from some of the girls was that not only are
you a midwife, you are also a social worker, a counsellor and a friend to
these women. Some of the girls didn't realise just how involved the midwife
was with the women within their remit. Being involved in a woman's care
who was expecting a baby with Down's syndrome, I can say that midwifery
is not only about 'catching babies' but there are sometimes 'bad' points
which show that midwifery isn't always roses.

The experience

Needless to say, a relationship of mutual trust and respect and sound
communication between the woman and her midwife is crucial to
achieving holistic woman-centred midwifery care and partnership,
which is the essence of midwifery. Putting the woman and her family
first is the most important part of the process, and relating to,
supporting and communicating with them make practising
midwifery worthwhile. This can be very rewarding for the woman
as well as the midwife and is very well illustrated in the following
impressions of a woman and her midwife:

Having total confidence in your midwife is so important. From the moment
onward that I met her [the midwife] all worries were taken away from
me and my midwife was superb in helping me and [reassuring] me. The
solid foundation of our relationship blossomed and the experience was
great. Three months after the birth of our baby, I can say the experience
still moves me. To find that special true congruent someone who takes
natural and extremely good care of you and when you most need it is of
paramount importance. The end of this story is really the beginning of
another, a story I cannot yet tell. This will no doubt benefit predominantly
my children and everyone around me on a daily basis.

I gain great pleasure working with women and their families ensuring that
holistic care is given at all times, which is imperative in midwifery. I always
hold close to me that pregnancy and childbirth is a lifetime experience that
women will remember and talk about forever and for myself to be part of
that memory and experience is very rewarding as well as overwhelming.

(Anglia Ruskin University 2008)

Conclusion

The word *midwife* means 'with women' or 'among women', sharing women's worries, their joys and their delights. To be a midwife is to engage in a close and intimate relationship, starting in pregnancy, with the effects travelling down through the centuries in the image women have of themselves, their abilities and their worth. Midwives and women are intertwined; whatever affects women affects midwives – women and midwives are interrelated and interwoven (Flint 1986, cited in Leap 2004). It is such intertwining that inspired me to become a midwife and has kept that enthusiasm going for over 15 years.

Commentary

Having worked as an independent midwife in the Netherlands, Yvonne is well placed to talk about the concept of normality experienced by most women during their pregnancies and discuss the midwife's role in relation to this. She cautions that, while this is the norm, the midwife needs to be vigilant and, if things deviate from the norm, appropriate referral needs to be made.

Yvonne also highlights the importance of partnership between the midwife and the woman. This concept is now well established, but it is important to note that it was not discussed in the literature prior to the late 1980s. Now it is shown that, working in a partnership, women and midwives can make decisions that will lead to the most appropriate and flexible package of care being provided.

Yvonne also draws on her experience of working with students and other midwives and uses their voices to enrich the chapter. Together, these voices reflect the importance of the midwife in contributing to the antenatal period, which is a time of change for the woman and the new family.

References

Anglia Ruskin University (2008) 'New generation midwife enhances birthing experience', *News and Events*, Cambridge and Chelmsford: Anglia Ruskin University.

International Confederation of Midwives (ICM) (2002) *Essential Competencies for Basic Midwifery Practice*, The Hague: ICM.

International Confederation of Midwives (ICM) (2005) *Definition of the Midwife*,The Hague: ICM.

Leap, N. (2004). 'Journey to midwifery through feminism: a personal account', in Stewart, M. (ed.) *Pregnancy, Birth and Maternity Care: Feminist perspectives*, London: Elsevier Butterworth Heinemann, pp. 185-200.

Leap, N. and Homer, C. (2002) 'A strategy to teach midwifery students about woman centred care in Australia', in Leap, N., Barclay, L., Brodie, P., Nagy, E., Sheehan, A. and Tracy, S. (eds) *National Review of Nursing Education: Midwifery education. Final Report, March 2002*, Sydney: Department of Education, Science and Training.

Walsh, D. and Steen, M. (2007) 'The role of the midwife: time for a review', *Midwives* 10(7): 320–3.

Chapter 2

Midwifery care with the woman in labour in an institution

Miranda Page

People are always fascinated when I say I am a midwife and yet very few ask me why I became one. Maybe that's a good thing, because I always feel my answer would disappoint; I would like to say that it's a career I have always wanted to do; that it was a calling, a need to be in touch with the life force or some divine inspiration. Well OK, maybe the last one is going a bit far. But anyway something serious and meditated, after careful consideration. You get the picture.

However, the long and the short of it is that it all happened on a Caledonian MacBrayne (CalMac to the locals) ferry from Mull to Oban. I had spent the last three years pondering life on a little island off Mull, drawing up lists of possible jobs following my abandonment of my previous life in London. Harrods, actually. But that's another story. And, I have to say, by that fateful trip for the monthly groceries, I hadn't come up with much.

The sad thing is I can't even remember her name, so I shall never be able to thank her. She was wearing dungarees, a big stripy hand-knitted jumper and bright red Doc Marten's. Pretty much standard dress for the inner Hebrides on a cold wet March morning. She was eating a bacon roll and drinking tea from a large white mug, which impressed me given the pitch and toss of the boat. 'A strong stomach' I thought, as I made to pass, heading for deck and fresh air. But I didn't pass; as I came level I was caught by . . . well . . . what was I caught by? It was the way she was talking, more than what she was saying. She was lit up. I found myself listening. No longer on the CalMac ferry but transported to a labour room, as she described the first birth she had ever seen as a student midwife. It was spell-binding. It was full of warmth and wit and a fair bit of drama. The way she described the woman, her partner and the midwife all working together to help this tiny wee baby come into the world was sheer magic. I remember thinking 'I could do with a bit of that magic in my life.' So, being a sucker for a good story, midwifery went to the top of my very short list of career options. And, as they say, 'the rest is history'.

Having had to reflect on my reasons for coming into midwifery for this chapter, it seems to me that what attracted me was this sense of togetherness, of working towards a common goal. Although the job did not turn out to be anything like I had expected, the one thing that kept me going was this sense of team working.

The theme of this chapter is midwifery care with the woman in labour in an institution. Given that this could be an entire book, I have concentrated on what I know best, namely team working and how it functions within an institution. There are many permutations of teams and members within each team. For this story I am concentrating on two:

1   The first team and probably the most central, though often forgotten, is one of midwives, women and their families. And, believe it or not, this is the main team that most midwives will work in. But where it might differ from other areas of midwifery practice is the number and different types of people that the midwife will come in contact with. Typically in any one shift, especially in large urban obstetric units, a midwife will be caring for a number of labouring women. She will be working alongside a number of midwives, not forgetting clinical support workers, and have contact with a multitude of birthing partners, husbands, grannies, aunties and Uncle Tom Cobleigh and all.

2   The second team involves the medical staff, midwives, the woman, and her partner and family. This team comes to the

fore either in emergencies or while caring for women with medical or obstetric complications. As above, in a typical labour ward there isn't just one member of each profession represented in the team. The midwife will usually liaise with a range of obstetricians, but can, especially in complicated cases, work with a range of other medical specialists, such as anaesthetists, neonatologists, diabetologists, haematologists, and even cardiologists!. Not something I ever expected to do when I was on that ferry to Oban.

The story told in this chapter comes largely from my own experience of working in a busy urban obstetric unit, but I have also drawn on an amalgam of events and characters conjured into being though the tales of labour ward life told to me at conferences, study days and workshops, at various times in my career as a practising midwife, RCM steward and researcher. I hope, therefore, that the midwives and events I describe will ring bells and provide food for thought for practising midwives in many settings, and, for those preparing to enter the profession, an insight into hospital life through the eyes of one midwife on a typical labour ward shift.

Midwifery and birthing babies

The shift started like any other, with me in the changing rooms donning the ubiquitous hospital scrubs, which invariably were either too small or too big. Today I had a top that could've hidden an elephant and a pair of bottoms belonging to a catwalk model. Still, at least I had a pair, matching or otherwise. Ruth, my colleague, wasn't having such luck and, despite going from pleading through bribing to offering to inflict bodily harm on people in the changing room, she was forced to admit defeat. As I headed to the labour ward I saw her heading to the postnatal ward to hunt down a pair of scrubs.

This particular day I was coordinating the shift. Twelve hours at the helm steering our way through hopefully calm waters with a motley crew and a precious cargo of mothers to be, new mums and babies and a few significant others thrown in for good measure.

Sue had been coordinating the night shift and, as I came through the doors, she turned her pale face towards me and smiled. Still huddled in her big woolly cardigan, she took one last sip of her now cold tea and walked with me to the duty room for report. I said a small prayer and promised that today would be different: 'Each woman that comes through that door will receive the best care. She will be valued and respected as a individual and her voice will be listened to.'

'Right hit me with it, Sue.'

'Well,' she said, taking a deep breath and looking at the board. 'You've got three normal labourers, two inductions, one on synto, the other one's waiting for an ARM but the head's high, a forceps in theatre, a possible pre-term labourer in room 4, one in HDU with a PPH, a diabetic in room 6, two delivered in 4 and 3. But postnatal's full, so God knows where you're going to put them.' A pause, 'Oh yes, and you've got 2 electives due and Alice has phoned in sick again.'

'Perfect,' I sighed.

'Here's the keys.' Sue thrust a large bundle of assorted metal into my hands. 'God, I nearly forgot, you'll have to order some more morphine; we've only got ten left.' With that she picked up her bag and hurried to the door. Turning round as her hand went to the handle, she smiled again and, with thoughts of a warm bed, waved goodbye.

As she left, the motley crew arrived. Through the duty room door came the day shift – all seven of them.

'Hold on a minute,' I thought . . . 'I know Alice is off sick but that still leaves us short by two.' I cast my eyes down the staff rota. 'Where's Sam and Joan?' I demanded. 'Study day,' someone muttered from the corner.

'Who said they could go on a bloody study day?'

'You did mate,' an Antipodean voice replied. I looked up, as rushing through the door in a mismatch of pink and orange came Ruth.

'Oh bugger, yes. Still, could be worse,' I reflected. 'You've found some 'blues' then?' Martha the student midwife smirked at the back. Ruth looked on defiantly.

'Okay team,' I said, trying to put a brave face on it. 'This is going to be a bit tricky, but I'm sure we can cope with whatever's thrown at us.'

'Struth, Miranda,' Ruth exclaimed as she chewed on a breakfast roll and looked at the board. Much as I enjoyed working with this laid-back funny New Zealander, sometimes, just sometimes, I wished she would engage her brain before she opened her mouth. I shot her a 'don't frighten the juniors look' and continued to rally the troops.

'This is what we are going to do. Who's working with Martha and Heather today?' The two student midwives looked distinctly nervous at the back of the room.

'It's Jane and me.' Jane was a keen young midwife, and the 'me' was Kristy. Kristy, the labour ward Mum. Every hospital should have one. She came with the bricks and had birthed just about the whole of the county as well as five of her own. At 55 she was as wide as she was tall, a bundle of warmth and tall stories, with a large bosom who had comforted and encouraged a whole generation of midwives and doctors. And she made the meanest chocolate cake in the whole world. The two students looked relieved. In fact, we all felt better having her on shift.

'OK then, why don't you and Jane take the normal labourers and the induction in room 5?' I said brightly.

Kristy froze, narrowed her eyes and rose to her full 4 foot 11 inches and said 'Not me, duck. Me, Jane and the girls will look after . . .' and then, turning to the board, she named the women in rooms 1, 2, 3 and 4. Ruth arched an eyebrow but didn't say anything because Kristy was right. And my mantra was in tatters and we were only half an hour into the shift. Duly chastened, I resolved to do better and allocated the rest of the staff to women, not conditions.

Jo was the last to leave and she did so rather reluctantly. I knew why. I had allocated her Mrs Jones, who was in early labour and a diabetic. Now Jo was a very good midwife, but she just didn't believe in herself. She got flustered very easily and lacked confidence. A woman with complicated needs would be challenging, but I knew with support she could do it. I tried to convey this to her, but going by her mournful expression as she walked down the corridor I hadn't succeeded.

'Just come and ask me if you're worried about anything,' I called after her retreating back. Her shoulders slumped even further. Well, I had enough to worry about – trying to find postnatal beds for the women who had already had their babies and the ward round to prepare for. Was this really what I had come into midwifery to do?

'Here, doll, get this down you!' Ruth pressed a steaming mug of tea into my hand as Lucy appeared with a tray of toast.

'It could be worse,' Lucy speculated. She would say that. I don't think I'd ever seen her ruffled. Not even the day when she had three sets of twins all deciding to be born at the same time!

'How could it be worse Lucy?'

'Well,' she paused as she took a bite of buttery toast. 'You see, you're really lucky – you've got the A team working today.'

I smiled, 'But who's Mr T?'

'Mr who?' came a perky voice from behind us.

'Sweetie, you're too young to remember,' Lucy said, turning to a rather excited Jane who was practically hopping from foot to foot. 'Oh right, whatever.' Frowning, she continued, 'just popped out to let you know that room 4's starting to push.'

'You mean,' said Ruth rather ominously waving an amni-hook in Jane's direction, 'Cynthia Patterson in room 4 is feeling the urge to bear down' and, turning to us with a 'See you later girls', she made her way into her own room still, I might add, waving her amni-hook.

'Well, that's what I meant,' said the rather surprised Jane. 'Ah well,' but before Lucy could launch forth a loud moan emanated from room 4 followed by the startled face of Martha, the student midwife.

'I think you might be wanted,' I pointed to Martha.

'Oh help,' Jane muttered and walked quickly to the door.

It shut as the dulcet tones of Cynthia Patterson rang out with 'There's no f**king way ya gonna get me to push . . . ohhhh ya bastard.'

'My, my and her a solicitor too,' commented Lucy as she went to answer the phone.

'Good morning, labour ward, Lucy Staples speaking . . . Jennifer who? . . . hold on . . . .' Placing her hand over the receiver, she lent over to me and whispered, 'How's room 3 doing? It's her mum,' nodding her head at the phone.

'Room 3 . . . room 3 . . . umm . . . yes . . . Let me go and check. That's Kristy's lady, hold on.' I walked down the corridor and knocked on the door.

'Hold on . . . with you in a tick,' came the reply. I stood and thought about the million other things I should be doing rather than waiting for Kristy and tried to breathe calmly. After what seemed an age the door was flung open.

'Aye up, me duck?'

'It's her mum wants to know how she's doing,' I said by way of a reply . . .

'Doing . . . well that all depends.'

'Yes, yes I know,' I sighed, instantly regretting my turn of phrase . . . 'but what can I tell her?'

Kristy looked down at her fob watch and ruminated. 'Tell her to call back at tea time.' 'Tea time!' I exclaimed. 'But . . .'. Kristy raised her left hand like a policeman stopping traffic. 'She's OP. I've put her in the bath. Teatime it will be.' And with that she turned and shut the door.

'Right you are,' I said under my breath and fast-footed it back to the phone where Lucy was looking at me expectantly.

'Tell her to call at tea time . . .'

'Hello, Mrs Adams,' said Lucy with her best telephone voice. 'The midwife looking after your daughter says to call again at tea time . . .'

'How long? . . .'

'Well, it's hard to tell . . .'

'Hopefully . . .'

'No, we can't give her something to speed it up . . .'

'Yes, I know it's been a long time . . .'

'Five days you say . . . well . . .'

'You had a drip . . . yes . . . well we try not to . . . uh uh . . .'

Lucy looked across at me and rolled her eyes.

'Just you call back at tea time and keep your fingers crossed,' she said and quickly put down the phone. It rang again straightaway we both stared at it and then each other. Taking a deep breath I picked it up. 'Good morning, labour ward, Miranda Page speaking . . .'

'Jennifer Adams . . . and you are . . .?'

'Her mother in law . . .'

'There's no news yet . . .'

'Yes. I know it does take time doesn't it . . . How long? Well it's hard to say . . .'

'Why don't you try phoning at tea time . . .?'

'Visiting . . . no not in labour ward . . . umm. I'm sorry, you'll have to wait until she goes to the postnatal ward . . .'

'So maybe you will be able to see her tomorrow . . .'

'Between 2 and 4 and 7 and 8 in the evening . . .'

'Well, that went down like a lead balloon . . .'

'Wanted to be at the delivery, did she?' Lucy asked.

'Yes. Would you really want your mother-in-law at the birth of your baby?'

'Can't think of anything worse, darling,' Lucy pondered, but her voice trailed off as the emergency buzzer in room 7 went off.

Lucy leapt to her feet and headed to the room. Two seconds later her head reappeared and she called, 'Fast bleep the paed would you. She's pushing and there's membranes visible – won't be long.'

I picked up the receiver and started to dial just as Jo moved into my line of vision, about to ask me a question. 'Give us a sec, Jo.'

'I just wanted to ask . . .'

'Yea, yea. Hold on . . .'. Answering the operator on the other end of the line, I said 'We need a paediatric registrar to labour ward, please. Thanks.' Hanging up, I said 'Sorry about that what did you . . .?' But I never got to finish the sentence because the phone rang again and it was admissions saying they had a woman coming up to labour ward pushing . . .

'Jo do us a favour run into room 9 and see if Mary can come out and look after this woman. Tell her she's going into room . . . God, do I have a room?'

I looked about wildly in the hope that an empty room would materialise in front of me like the Tardis. It didn't, but what did was Leila, our godsend of a clinical support worker, walking beside Anne Thompson from room 8. Anne, as proud as punch carrying her new baby. Dad on the other side as white as a sheet. Trailing behind was mum. I know we are only supposed to have one partner per room but sometimes it's hard to say 'No'.

As the new family tottered down the corridor I heard Anne's mum saying to Leila, 'Well, she was a bit flat at birth. But you know the midwife just took her outside and pumped her up and now look, she's just fine; it's the happiest day of my life.' At which point she burst into tears. And off they went, barely missing the paed belting down the corridor towards them.

'What room?' he bellowed.

'7'

'Which one's that?'

I refrained from saying 'It's the one next to 6' and pointed behind him. 'That one.'

'Great.' Checking his stethoscope, which was threatening to wrap itself around his throat, he smoothed his hair down and calmly walked into the room. 'Hello there! I'm Dr Jenkins the paediatrician . . .'

Just when you think it can't get any worse, the lady from admissions appeared in a wheelchair, puffing madly . . .

'I told you we didn't have time to wait for the end of the football,' she exclaimed, whacking her husband in the chest with her handheld notes.

'Where do you want her, love?' asked the ambulance driver.

Praying that the room was clean, 'room 8,' I replied, waving vaguely in its direction. And just when you really, really don't need it – in walked the ward round.

What can you say about the ward round? It is an institution and its daily occurrence is played out in just about every obstetric labour ward in the UK. Probably in much the same way and at the same time. The entourage consisted of Dr Munroe, consultant obstetrician and soon to be Professor of Obs and Gyne, thus head honcho, surrounded by a gaggle of registrars, senior house officers (SHOs) and medical students. In all, nine more bodies cluttering up the narrow corridor that acted as the major artery running through the labour ward, which right now was in danger of bursting at the seams.

'Sister, good morning to you! And what have you got for us this morning?' He stood rubbing his hands together and rocking back and forth. Old school. No one else called me sister – what was I, a nun! He was a big man of slightly rotund build. Shall we say? And he was looking at me in anticipation. He raised an eyebrow as I was about to launch forth. I hesitated as I caught, out of the corner of my eye, the fleeting figure of May Chen, our anaesthetist, bustling towards room 2. Must be for an epidural, I surmised . . . oh well . . . yes, yes, what was I saying? Dr Munroe coughed to draw my attention back to the task at hand. While I was trying to put my brain into gear, we headed to the high-dependency unit (HDU) and our lady with the PPH. 'Right, today we have Sheila Miller, a 31-year-old multigravida . . .'. For the next half an hour I was preoccupied with describing the women we had in the labour ward and their many complications.

The entourage made its way around the labour ward, stopping at various rooms, where they prodded and poked, offering reassurance and dispensing advice. In between the rooms, Dr Munroe quizzed the medical students about the conditions they had just seen.

When we arrived at Jo's room, I was relieved to see her looking a little less frazzled. But I was also struck with guilt as I remembered she had been desperate to ask me something. I looked at her, trying to convey an apology. 'Did you manage to get some help?' I mouthed, as Dr Munroe, the registrars, SHOs and medical students squeezed into the room. Was it really possible to get 13 people into one tiny labour room, and that's including the poor woman and her partner? Oh, and Ruth.

Ruth was bending over one of the many pumps attached to Cath Wright, our 'diabetic'. 'That should do you now,' she said, tapping on the screen at the front of the contraption.

'Thanks so much.' Jo heaved a sigh of relief.

'No worries. Onwards and upwards, and while you're here,' Ruth said, turning her attention to 'the posse', as she liked to call the ward round. 'You don't need to come to my room. We're doing absolutely fine. I'll give you a shout if we need you . . . OK mate?' she ended, directing her gaze at the soon-to-be Prof.

'Absolutely . . . right sister . . . of course.'

Ruth exited the room, but I distinctly heard her muttering, 'Do I look like a bleeding nun?'

I left the group with Jo giving an update on Cath Wright's progress and popped my head out into the corridor. You never know what might happen when your back's turned. All seemed remarkably quiet. The faint whiff of toast lingered in the air, a sign that a baby had just arrived. It mingled with the smell of disinfectant and the distinct aroma of boiled cabbage. You can't beat that hospital smell. The sun must have been shining, as the afterglow of light filtered through the glass panel of the sluice door − the only light that reached the labour ward corridor. Footsteps echoed around the corner and the slow grating metal on metal of an erratic trolley added to the eerie air of calm.

A small 'ping ping bong' sound caught my attention. I saw the door of room 7 open and, coming out, pushed by the paed, an incubator with our latest arrival going to the neonatal unit around the corner. It was closely followed by dad clutching a mobile and a sheet of paper with a list of names to phone. He looked rather shaken but smiled at me as he passed.

'Four pounds,' he said in amazement. 'Thanks so much.'

The day progressed in much the same way. Jo cheered up and she looked positively happy when I saw her ensconced in the treatment room with our new registrar, calculating Cath's insulin regime. Nice to see doctors and midwives working so well together, I thought in passing.

By teatime, Lucy and I were back at the desk surveying the damage. We had just about cleared the board by 5 o'clock, but it was beginning, as always, to fill up again. Jane had had three deliveries and was sitting resting her feet, while Martha, her student, was eyeing up the box of chocolates that lay unopened on the desk.

'Go on, open them! You know you want to,' Jane said as the phone rang. Lucy stretched a rather weary arm out.
'Labour ward. Lucy Staples speaking. How can I help?'
She looked up at me and nodded towards Kristy's room. 'Any news yet?'
'I'll just go and check.' Finding it rather difficult to rouse myself, I moved from my chair and wandered down the corridor. Heather answered the door. Behind her shoulder I could see the huddled shapes of Sarah Adams, still in the pool, her baby snuggled into her chest and dad kneeling behind with his arms around them both. They were cocooned in a velvety light washed over by soft music. I could just make out Kristy sitting in a rocking chair – peacefully filling in her notes. She looked up and smiled. Giving Heather the thumbs up, I gently closed the door. Coming back to the desk, I said to Lucy 'Tell her that someone will be phoning very shortly.'

So that was that really. A typical day for us, but one of the most memorable and special for the women we were caring for. Just before 8 p.m. the door opened and Sue walked in.
'All right girls,' she said. I picked up the keys to make my way to the duty room after her. 'Oh God,' I yelped, making everyone jump. 'The morphine. I've forgot to order the ruddy morphine . . .'
It's Okay doll. I did it this afternoon.'
'Ruth, I could kiss you.'
'Steady on mate.'

Team working

There has been much said about labour ward cultures and professional and group dynamics. Too much to go into here. For further reading in midwifery, look at the works of Mavis Kirkham (1999), Nicky Leap (1997), Tina Lavender and Jean Chapple (2004) and Belinda Green (2005). In the field of health care sociology, I would suggest the works of Keith Macdonald (1995), Louise Fitzgerald et al. (2003) and David Buchanan et al. (2005) to get a flavour of team working and its many complexities.

What resonates most with me, however, is the work done by Billie Hunter (2004, 2005) and Rosalind Bluff (2001). Hunter describes the many difficulties faced by midwives, particularly coping with the demands of the women they care for, while also keeping an eye out for the expectations and demands of the hospital unit, their managers and colleagues – the 'being with woman or with institution'.

In Bluff's work, she describes the different ways midwives interpret and use 'rules'. These 'rules' are set by the team. If there is conflict within the team as to what constitutes the 'rules' (the midwifery versus medical model springs to mind), midwives will adopt different strategies to apply the 'rules' they are most comfortable with. Hence, 'the prescriptive or flexible midwife'.

Their research and my own experience seems to demonstrate that, for the hospital midwife, 'the team' encompasses more than just the midwife and the woman. It goes further and involves a multitude of players, be they medical, midwifery or the woman's own family.

I hope this story has demonstrated that having a team that works well is not an easy feat. Its creation utilises a combination of skill, art and science, although I have known midwives who make it look like child's play. Its success or failure can be gauged by the quality of care women receive on any one shift. To achieve this, the team must function effectively on a number of levels. By that I mean an effective team needs the right skill mix, adequate staffing levels and the ability to communicate effectively, not only between its members, but also with the women they care for. For me, however, the most important quality a team needs is the ability to support each other, not only on professional matters, but also emotionally with the everyday, and not so everyday, stresses of working in a busy unit.

So what does this all add up to? I wanted to go into midwifery because of the description of birth I heard on that CalMac ferry: 'The woman, her partner and the midwife all working together to help this tiny wee baby come into the world was sheer magic.'

It seems to me that what I did was work in the plural. Instead of being involved in helping that one woman and that one baby, I created, as best I could with the resources available, the environment that helped lots of mothers have lots of babies with hopefully lots of midwives all experiencing that 'bit of magic'. It wasn't easy and I didn't always manage to pull it off, but I tried, as we all do every day.

Commentary

In spite of her apparently light-hearted approach, Miranda's chapter illuminates the seriously complex role of the midwife working in a labour ward. This midwife is not just required to be 'with woman' and 'with institution'; she also carries responsibility for ensuring the effective functioning of the clinical area. This observation resonates with the findings of a number of researchers who have explored the role of the midwife in this context, most recently Keating and Fleming (2008). These research findings demonstrate the convoluted strategies that this midwife must adopt to maintain both her or his own integrity and the satisfaction of the women giving birth in the labour ward. As has been shown previously by Kitzinger et al. (1990), midwives are forced to resort to a wide range of strategies and tactics to achieve the positive outcomes that childbearing women deserve.

Kitzinger et al. identified the communicative or manipulative skills the midwife needs in order to persuade junior medical staff to act, or perhaps intervene, appropriately. The smooth running of the labour ward depends on such communication skills, but they must be employed surreptitiously: 'You just have to make them feel important and learn how to pull the right strings' (1990: 156).

Whereas I might use the term 'feminine wiles' to explain such activity, and Mary Cronk has dubbed it 'doing good by stealth', Kitzinger et al. labelled it 'hierarchy maintenance work'. On the basis of these labels and this behaviour, we may need to question the professional status of the midwife.

References

Bluff, R. (2001) 'Learning and teaching in the context of clinical practice: the midwife as role model', unpublished Ph.D. thesis, Bournemouth University.

Buchanan, D., Fitzgerald, L., Ketley, D. and Gollop, R. et al. (2005) 'No going back: a review of the literature on sustaining organizational change', International Journal of Management Reviews 7(3): 189–205.

Fitzgerald, L., Ferlie, E. and Hawkins, C. (2003) 'Innovations in healthcare: how does creditable evidence influence professionals?' *Health and Social Care in the Community* 11(3): 219–28.

Green, B. (2005) 'Midwives' coping methods for managing birth uncertainties', *British Journal of Midwifery* 13(5): 293–8.

Hunter, B. (2004) 'Conflicting ideologies as a source of emotion work in midwifery', *Midwifery* 20: 261–72.

Hunter, B. (2005) 'Emotion work and boundary maintenance in hospital-based midwifery' *Midwifery* 21: 253–66.

Keating, A. and Fleming, V.E.M. (2008) 'Midwives' experiences of facilitating normal birth in an obstetric-led unit: a feminist perspective', *Midwifery*, 25 January. Available online, reference doi:10.1016/j.midw.2007.08.009.

Kirkham, M. (1999) 'The culture of midwifery in the National Health Service in England', *The Journal of Advanced Nursing* 30(3): 732–9.

Kitzinger J., Green J. and Coupland V. (1990) 'Labour relations: midwives and doctors on the labour ward', in Garcia J., Kilpatrick R. and Richards, M. (eds) *The Politics of Maternity Care: Services for childbearing women in 20th century Britain*, Oxford: Clarendon Press, pp. 149–62.

Lavender, T. and Chapple, J. (2004) 'An exploration of midwives' views of the current system of maternity care', *Midwifery* 20: 324–34.

Leap, N. (1997) 'Birthwrite. Making sense of 'horizontal violence' in midwifery', *British Journal of Midwifery* 5(11): 689.

Macdonald, K.M. (1995) *The Sociology of the Professions*, London: Sage.

Chapter 3

Midwifery care of the mother and baby at home

Allison Ewing

It is now 26 years since I embarked on my journey to be a midwife. As a student nurse in 1984, I saw that first-time mothers were kept in hospital for the full statutory ten days! This seems astonishing now, but was necessary as there were not enough midwives to provide community postnatal care. The district nurses were 'double duty' and didn't have enough time to provide both nursing and midwifery care. Mothers on subsequent pregnancies were 'allowed' out after four days. Fortunately, this did appear to give the women a good grounding in breastfeeding and basic baby care before they went home.

The role of the midwife in the community postnatally may have been idealised. Given the above vignette, it can be seen that this is not always true as, even then, community postnatal care was seen as the Cinderella service of maternity care. Because of this, I became a community midwife in order to provide a holistic continuity of midwifery care from antenatal through home birth to postnatal care. This crystalised after I attended my first home birth as a student midwife. I have likened this to my Damascene conversion! But that was 22 years ago. In many areas now, women are being told that they can't have a home birth as there will not be a midwife available to come out to them when they go into labour even if they have booked a home birth.

This chapter will address the issue of postnatal care of the mother and baby in the home environment. It will look at the historical basis for and practice of midwifery care at home and at what has become of postnatal care at home in the twenty-first century, then go on to detail a wish list for postnatal care.

The historical basis of community-based postnatal care

What is, or was, postnatal care? When midwifery care was regulated at the beginning of the twentieth century, one of the main causes of mortality and morbidity of women and babies was either maternal or neonatal sepsis. Until 1986, there was a statutory requirement in the *Midwives Rules* for midwives to visit the woman daily until ten days postpartum, with a recommendation that the woman have two visits a day in the first few days if she had given birth at home (Sweet 1983; Garcia *et al.* 1994). In the tenth edition of *Mayes' Midwifery* (Sweet 1983), the chapter on postnatal complications is mostly concerned with the detection, by the midwife, of postnatal infections in the mother and in the baby.

The midwife would, therefore, be regularly taking the pulse and temperature of the postnatal woman to assess if there was a developing fever. She would be assessing the breasts and nipples for any sign of trauma from breastfeeding, as this could lead to mastitis and breast abscess. She would enquire about vaginal discharge (lochia) for colour, odour and amount. In 'top to toe' examination she would then be palpating the uterus to detect if it was involuting (returning to its normal size and location in the pelvic cavity) and whether it was tender to the touch. Next might be a question about passing urine and opening bowels. Urinary tract infection might be a risk, as there is dilatation of the ureters in pregnancy and the woman may have difficulty in fully emptying her bladder. This can result in some urine remaining in the urinary tract, allowing bacteria to grow. The woman might also be reluctant to pass urine if she has grazes or suffers other trauma to the genital area. Her perineum would be inspected, if she had sustained damage to it, to assess healing. Finally, she would be asked about her legs, as there would be a perceived risk of thromboembolism. This is because, after the birth, the blood becomes more viscous again as the excess fluid that has been in the cardiovascular system in pregnancy is excreted soon after the baby is born. Women with a previous history of varicose veins would be more at risk. Thromboembolism was also probably more prevalent as a result of the advice for the woman to be nursed in bed.

The midwife would then turn her attention to the baby. Sleeping, feeding and excreting habits would be enquired about. She might then perform a 'top to toe' examination to assess the colour of the baby (looking for jaundice) and tone. She would be looking at the eyes, mouth, skin and umbilicus for signs of infection, as in the mother. For the midwife then, 'cleanliness was next to Godliness' and great care was to be taken to prevent infection with thorough handwashing most important (Sweet 1983).

If this was a first-time mother, the midwife might then demonstrate how to 'top and tail' the baby and bath the baby, give breast-feeding support or show how to make up a bottle feed safely. One advantage that the midwife and mother had was that they would likely know each other, as there was a good chance that the midwife would have provided the antenatal care as well as being present at the birth.

Very little is written in Sweet (1983) about the emotional and mental well-being of the mother, with only two pages devoted to 'Psychiatric Disorders'. On page 413 can be found the following:

> A calm and placid woman, happily married and secure, may weather the emotional storms of pregnancy, labour and the puerperium without more than an occasional attack of 'blues'. One who is temperamentally more anxious and nervous may find the same degree of emotional strain intolerable. For the woman with a history of mental instability the stress of pregnancy and labour may initiate a recurrence of mental illness.

This is in marked contrast to, 20 years later, the detailed chapter in the fourteenth edition of the *Myles Textbook for Midwives* (Fraser and Cooper 2003), which addresses this issue, also discussed in more detail in Chapter 4 of this book.

In the mid part of the twentieth century, the community midwife was seen as a valued and integral part of the community. Worth (2007) and Joyce (2008) have both written vivid and moving memoirs of midwifery care in the 1950s and 1960s. It is not altogether a rosy picture and there was a great deal of poverty and deprivation in the areas in which they worked; the work depicted was demanding and hard. The community midwife in those times was usually also a Midwifery Sister and would have a higher salary than most of her hospital counterparts to reflect the greater clinical responsibility in attending 'home confinements'.

After the Peel Report in 1970 and the recommendation that *all* births should be in hospital, the role of the community midwife was vastly reduced to consist mostly of staffing antenatal clinics and performing postnatal visits. The de-skilling of midwives who could attend home births continued. At this time it would be highly unlikely that a midwife would be attending a woman she knew in labour, although there might be good continuity of care and carer in the ante- and postnatal periods.

In the late 1980s and early 1990s, there was a resurgence in midwives trying to reclaim midwifery in the community with initiatives such as the Know Your Midwife scheme, founded by Caroline Flint, and the One To One scheme, instigated by Lesley Page. Both of these projects were attempting to provide more continuity of care and carer in the whole of the pregnancy, labour and postnatal period (Page 2003).

With the Flint scheme, the aim was that the woman would have met the midwife attending her in labour at least once in the antenatal period. I was fortunate to work in the first NHS roll-out of this scheme in the early 1990s, being in a team of six midwives who were all earning the same salary. It was an exciting time to be working and was manageable when there was a realistic caseload for the team and the team was of a small enough size for effective communication and cooperation. There was great job satisfaction as a midwife, but a mother might have felt that there was less continuity of carer in the postnatal period, as all members of the team took it in turns to staff the antenatal clinics, be on call for labour and perform the postnatal visits. The team ran coffee mornings for groups of women due in the same month, so that they could meet each other and the team.

The Page One to One scheme has now become known as Caseload Midwifery and, for many midwives and mothers, this can provide the ideal way to work and be cared for. For this to work, though, there has to be a realistic caseload. This will be discussed more in the next section.

That was then, this is now

So how have things changed? What are the challenges facing the average community midwife today? Sadly, the remit for community-based midwives remains the same, although they are working in a much more pressured environment.

I would say that one of the biggest challenges to the modern community midwife now is that there are not enough of them to go round. There is a recognised shortage of midwives in many parts of the UK. Numbers are debated by Government and the Royal College of Midwives (RCM), but the reality is that there are fewer Whole Time Equivalent Midwives (WTEs) than there were 20 years ago. The introduction of more family-friendly employment policies, and parity of pay and conditions between part-time and full-time workers, has encouraged more midwives, especially those with young families, to work part-time,. Also, some midwives without children might simply choose to work part-time to relieve stress at work. So, while numbers of midwives might look the same on paper, there are still too few WTEs.

As maternity services are centralised, the concentration of births in the large Obstetric Units has also meant that, when there is a shortage of midwives, the remaining ones will need to be concentrated in the high-risk and potentially litigious area of intrapartum care.

So where does that leave community postnatal care, if most of the midwives are in the hospital?

After the ten-day statutory requirement was removed in the 1980s, selective visiting slowly became the norm. Part of the rationale for the removal of the statutory requirement was that, in some cases, midwives were visiting some women who were not at home and thus not seen to be in need of midwifery services. This was obviously a waste of the midwives' time and the NHS's money. The introduction of selective visiting was supposed to be in partnership and agreement with the needs of the mother and was generally welcomed by midwives.

In many cases, it started with the woman being visited daily for approximately the first four days and then on alternative days until day 10, when care would be handed over to the health visitor. The *Midwives Rules* still maintained that a midwife could visit up to 28 days, but the midwife would have to demonstrate a good reason why a woman might still be 'on the books' after ten days. Her time-management skills might be called into question if she couldn't manage to see 12 postnatal women and run a two-hour antenatal clinic in an eight-hour day.

It is deeply depressing to report that this slippery slope to the erosion of midwifery postnatal care has become an even steeper incline. In many places in England where the midwifery shortage has bitten deep, many women are only getting one or two visits in the ten-day period. This is despite the fact that hospitals with fewer beds than 20 years ago are having to discharge women as quickly as possible back into the community.

In this time it was expected that, between visits, the woman would be able to recognise if there were any problems with her or her baby and be able to contact a midwife if necessary. The one or two visits are functional to weigh the baby and to take the heel-prick test, which is essential to diagnose many metabolic disorders. That, unfortunately, is the sum of what many community midwives, due to pressure of work, are able to do in the postnatal period.

An example from the field showing some of the potential dangers

Sheila, an independent midwife, has attended the successful home birth of Jane. This is Jane's second birth with Sheila. Sheila has visited on days 1, 2, 3 and 5. On day 5 she weighs the baby and performs the heel-prick test. She has practised selective visiting, but this woman is an experienced mother and the decision to miss out days has been a joint one. Now, in the current format of standard postnatal care in some areas, this might be when the visits by the midwife stop, but Sheila has the 'luxury' of being able to give more time and individualised care to Jane and her baby and arranges to come back on day 7. The baby has been slightly jaundiced, but not enough to interfere with breastfeeding or excretion. When the midwife returns on day 7, Jane reports that the baby has been more sleepy and reluctant to feed. The jaundice isn't any worse; in fact, if anything it looks better. The midwife can't put her finger on what is wrong with the baby. The baby's temperature is 37.5, heartbeat is 140 and respirations are 40. The woman's other child is off nursery that day with a respiratory virus. The midwife inspects the umbilicus: clean and healing with no sign of inflammation. She pulls down the nappy and there she finds a small 50p-sized lesion/blister just on the right groin, looking red and inflamed, with some pus in the centre. The mother hadn't noticed it being there when she had changed the nappy a couple of hours earlier. The midwife recommends that the baby be seen at the local children's hospital.

Jane waits for her husband to come home and goes to the hospital. The baby is admitted and has intravenous antibiotics for four days for scalded skin syndrome caused by staphylococcus aureus, which was beginning to become a systemic infection.

There are two questions I would like to ask:

1   What might have happened had that woman been having a standard visiting pattern?
2   She was an experienced mother and might have been expected to notice something like that. Why didn't she?

The baby was discharged on oral antibiotics after four days, had continued to breastfeed in hospital and luckily didn't get thrush as a result of taking the antibiotics. Sheila was able to continue to give care in tandem with the health visitor until she was satisfied that the baby was on the mend. Sheila did not fully discharge this mother and her baby from her care until day 32. He continues to thrive. It would seem that the role of the midwife in detecting postnatal infections might still be needed.

Unfortunately, some cases of postnatal infection are being missed or dismissed (BBC 2008). A midwife was struck off the NMC register in December 2008 for failing to spot that a woman was developing a septicaemia. The woman subsequently died. On reading the report and related articles, it transpires that the woman had been seen by two other midwives and a GP before being visited by the midwife in question. The midwife had been placed on 'conditions of practice' following the death of the mother, but had subsequently made more mistakes. The midwife's GP had made a statement that she had been suffering from post-traumatic stress disorder and depression during the period since the death.

More questions:

1   Would continuity of carer have had any effect on the outcome?
2   The midwife had also been a community midwife for many years. Without wanting to excuse her actions in any way, what changes in her working pattern may she have experienced in her working life? How much time were the midwives able to spend on the visits?

Despite this, the erosion of home-based postnatal care has been completed in Calcot near Newbury in Berkshire (Owen 2009). Here, the shortage of midwives must be so acute that the local Trust has now opened a drop-in centre in the local Sainsbury's so that women can bring their babies to be weighed! The facility is only open for babies between two and ten days old and mothers can book a 20-minute appointment to see a midwife. This is presented as a greatly convenient opportunity for busy new mothers. I have to admit that, on reading that, I had a mental picture of Maggie being scanned through the supermarket checkout in the opening credits of the well-known television series 'The Simpsons'!

This book has been aimed at prospective midwives. Many of you reading this may be mothers yourself. Would any of you have felt like taking your baby to a supermarket to be weighed in the first ten days after they were born? If you were feeling unwell, would you feel able to get yourself and your baby out to the supermarket or even a health centre drop-in postnatal clinic?

Another example illustrating the value of community-based postnatal care

Sheila has another client, Norma. The midwife sees her client at 35 weeks, two days before she is going on holiday for a week. The woman has been planning a home birth for her first baby, but the midwife will be back before the woman is term at 37 completed weeks of pregnancy.

The midwife has been at her destination for four hours before her mobile phone rings and the woman says that she thinks she is going into labour. As Norma is still only 35 weeks, Sheila has to advise that, even if she were not on holiday, she would still recommend that Norma have a hospital birth, as the baby would be slightly premature. After discussion with Norma, it is agreed that Sheila will remain on holiday as they both expect that mother and baby will remain in hospital for several days as the baby will be premature. Sheila arranges to come home from holiday a day early, hopefully to coincide with the hospital discharge. Norma proceeds to a quick 'normal' birth in hospital but is then, to the surprise of Sheila, discharged after only two days as 'they needed the bed'. The irony is that this is the same hospital that used to keep first-time mothers of term babies in for ten days!

Sheila has already contacted the local Link Supervisor of Midwives (SOM) before this and now contacts her again to request that community midwives provide initial postnatal care. This is agreed.

Two days after the discharge from hospital, the baby is readmitted from home with dehydration and jaundice. The baby is still in hospital when Sheila returns, but is discharged that day. Sheila then spends the next six days making daily visits to the family to support the breastfeeding (days 7 to 12). Unfortunately, this time there is no health visitor input as there is one off sick, one vacancy and one on holiday. Again, Sheila had the 'luxury' of being able to spend enough time with Norma to get the feeding established and the baby back to birth weight. She was also able to recognise and keep an eye on the fact that Norma was showing some early signs of slight depression.

This might have sounded like a criticism of individual midwives, but is a criticism of the system that forces them to work in unacceptable circumstances.

It is not all doom and gloom. There are pockets of excellent midwifery care all over the UK, but a lot of it seems to be in rural areas: Montrose, Powys, Torbay. If you live and work in an urban area, the chances are that the only option for you will be in a large centralised Obstetric Unit or two. Depending on where you live, you might have to serve your time in that large unit until judged experienced enough to be allowed out into the community. In another area, you might be able to become a caseload midwife almost as soon as you qualify. However, if you want to work in a caseload scheme, most, if not all, of them are in England or Wales.

Blue sky thinking or cloud cuckoo land?

The language used in the first section of this chapter was deliberately archaic and formal to reflect the teaching and expectations of the time. The twenty-first-century textbook now talks about the midwife helping in the transition and adaptation to parenthood and working in partnership with the woman (Marchant 2003). A lot more emphasis is now placed on the emotional and mental well-being of the mother, as well it should (Raynor and Oates 2003).

There is criticism that the 'top to toe' examination may not give the woman space to articulate her real concerns. However, in order for the woman to be able to do this, she is going to need time and some may need to feel comfortable with the midwife to be able to express themselves.

Towards the end of my time as a community midwife in the NHS, the time constraints were becoming tighter and I was spending less time on postnatal visits. It was frustrating to know that, if I wanted to get round all my visits, I would not want to find any 'problems' that would need action or take time. I did not always have the time to spend with a woman in order to assist in breastfeeding or to notice any clues that she might want to talk about anything.

I had been a midwife for six years before I became a mother and I have to confess that, until then, I had not truly appreciated the value of having community postnatal care. I was also doubly lucky in that I had been cared for by two of my friends and colleagues and had not truly appreciated the value of continuity of care and carer until that time. I am absolutely sure that my birth and my adaptation to motherhood would have been quite different had I experienced fragmented care. As an aside, in a nearby hospital, midwives are now banned from caring for colleagues, friends or relatives.

Marchant (2003) makes the observation that the British provision of community postnatal care is unique or unusual from an international perspective. In many countries, maternity care from an obstetrician or midwife stops as the woman walks out of the hospital door. She points out that it is only recently that America and Canada have started to introduce postpartum home visits and support programmes and that, in the Netherlands, most of the postnatal care is given by maternity aides.

But why should we wish to get rid of our unique service? Evans (2001) makes a passionate plea to retain and to 'fight for the protection of one of the jewels of the midwifery service in the UK' and I wholeheartedly agree with her.

In the end, it all comes down to cost. Postnatal services are the first to go when more cuts have to be made. Midwives are considered to be expensive, but would it surprise you to know that the wage of an average community midwife has not actually risen very much in the 12 years since I stopped being one? When I left in 1996, my wage as a top G Grade midwife, including London weighting and enhancements, was approximately £26,000. Seven years later, in 2003, a caseload midwife in Bristol was earning £26,340 (*Guardian* 2003). In the article, she reported that her caseload had increased and that she was feeling increasingly stressed and undervalued. After Agenda for Change in 2004, most surviving G Grade community midwives were put on Band 6, while the Gs in the hospital were given Band 7. Today, there is an advertisement for a Band 6 community midwife in London with a starting salary of £28,924 (*Guardian Jobs* 2009).

In these days of 'credit crunch' and belt-tightening, perhaps midwives will just need to be grateful they have a job, however stressful and undervalued. Perhaps it could be seen as crass to be talking about how much midwifery care is worth, when all around people are losing their jobs. However, the increase in stress and feeling undervalued may be having a direct impact on the care being provided, as seen in the case of the midwife in Wales (BBC 2008).

I make no apologies for taking a political stance. Words like 'pragmatic' and 'realistic' are used to justify the cost-cutting. Words like 'essential' and 'necessary' need to be adopted again to describe community postnatal care. I believe that the future health of mothers and their new families is too important and needs to be supported to the utmost. Don't forget, this is also the future health of the country.

Women and their midwives are going to have to fight very hard to reclaim the ground that has been lost.

Commentary

Allison speaks passionately about postnatal care as the Cinderella of the maternity services, a comment that resonates strongly with me. One of my earliest experiences of working in New Zealand was as night supervisor of a large (400 beds) obstetric and gynaecological hospital. To my amazement, the only other midwives were in labour ward and the antenatal ward with registered or enrolled nurses staffing the four postnatal wards.

It appears that the situation is not improving greatly for women and is frustrating for midwives who are supposed to, as Allison has pointed out, limit themselves to a short period of time for the provision of postnatal services. However, if time permits, providing postnatal care can be extremely rewarding for both mother and midwife. It is a time during which many changes are taking place and in which women, whether healthy or otherwise, are looking for guidance from experts. In the provision of services to women in the postnatal period, midwives are the experts and can give guidance or simply be available to listen and reinforce decisions that the woman makes.

Where things start to go wrong, as Allison has shown, midwives are those who recognise the problem and refer appropriately to other health professionals. The value of a good, observant midwife in the postnatal period therefore cannot be underestimated, and midwives need to fight to be able to retain some autonomy over their workload in this area, thus making it once more a valuable and rewarding career choice.

References

British Broadcasting Corporation (BBC) (2008) 'Midwife struck off after death', News Channel. Available online at http://news.bbc.co.uk/1/hi/wales/7775755.stm (accessed 12 January 2009).

Department of Health (DH) (1970) *The Peel Report*, London: HMSO.

Evans, J. (2001) 'Woman-centred postnatal care: the personal view of an independent midwife', *MIDIRS Midwifery Digest* 1 (suppl. 1, March): S7–S8.

Fraser, D.M and Cooper M.A. (eds) (2003) *Myles Textbook for Midwives*, 14th edition, Edinburgh: Churchill Livingstone.

Garcia, J., Renfrew, M. and Marchant, S. (1994) 'Postnatal home visiting by midwives', *Midwifery* 10(1), March: 40–3.

Guardian (2003) 'Community midwife, Bristol', *Public Voices: Public Values*. Available online at www.guardian.co.uk/society/2003/mar/s0/public voices27 (accessed 12 January 2009).

Guardian Jobs (2009) Available online at http://jobs.guardian.co.uk/job/802036/midwife-practitioners-band-6-midwifery-guys-and-st-thomas-nhs-foundation-trust/ (accessed 12 January 2009).

Joyce, H. (2008) *The Green Lady: Memoirs of a Glasgow midwife*, Canada: Circle 49 Publishing Association.

Marchant, S. (2003) 'The puerperium', in Fraser, D.M. and Cooper M.A. (eds) *Myles Textbook for Midwives*, 14th edition, Edinburgh: Churchill Livingstone.

Owen, P. (2009) 'A pint of milk and a health check for my baby, please'. Available online at www.newburytoday.co.uk/News/Article.aspx?articleID=8925 (accessed 12 January 2009).

Page, L. (2003) 'Woman-centred, midwife-friendly care: principles, patterns and culture of practice', in Fraser, D.M and Cooper M.A. (eds) *Myles Textbook for Midwives*, 14th edition, Edinburgh: Churchill Livingstone.

Raynor, M.D. and Oates, M.R. (2003) 'The psychology and psychopathology of pregnancy and childbirth', in Fraser, D.M and Cooper M.A. (eds) *Myles Textbook for Midwives*, 14th edition, Edinburgh: Churchill Livingstone.

Sweet, B.R. (ed.) (1983) *Mayes' Midwifery: A textbook for midwives*, 10th edition, London: Baillière Tindall.

Worth, J. (2007) *Call The Midwife: A true story of the East End in the 1950s*, London: Weidenfeld and Nicolson.

Chapter 4

Midwives and perinatal mental health

Eleanor Forrest

Emma's friend, Ros, has noticed that, since becoming pregnant, Emma has been very nervous and preoccupied. Emma is now 12 weeks pregnant. Ros talks with Emma, who confides that she is really worried about the baby. This is because Emma had a lot of alcohol to drink around the time she fell pregnant. Now Emma can't sleep properly, has difficulty concentrating and feels nervous all the time.

Although the exact reasons are not clear, we recognise that stress and anxiety in pregnancy can have adverse effects. These include premature labour, separation of the placenta, low infant birth weight and the baby being born in a poor condition. Pregnant women such as Emma experience similar anxieties and concerns, and mild to moderate levels of anxiety are common, and are linked with physical problems such as increased heart rate.

The above vignette is an example of a very common issue that a woman might mention to me, as her midwife. It does not mean that Emma has a mental health problem, but it might alert me to spend extra time with Emma discussing these issues further and arranging support if necessary.

The midwife and mental health

It is not easy to sum up the midwife's role, as it is very diverse. As you will have read in other chapters in this book, a midwife examines the woman, provides childbirth education and supports the woman and her family throughout the perinatal period. To do this effectively, the midwife also collaborates with other health and social care professionals to meet the specific needs of the mother. For example, as well as caring for those women whose pregnancy, birth and post-natal experience are relatively problem-free, the midwife also provides expert care for:

- the woman with mental health problems;
- the teenage mother;
- the mother who is socially excluded;
- the mother with a substance misuse problem;
- the woman living with domestic abuse;
- women from diverse ethnic backgrounds.

(RCM 2008)

Therefore, as you can perhaps see, consideration of the mental health of women in the perinatal period is only one aspect of a midwife's role; however, the importance of this is often misunderstood and underestimated (Price 2007). Although this topic can perhaps be discussed by considering some relevant issues of perinatal mental health that are pertinent to midwives and their public health role, within just one chapter I cannot thoroughly explore or justify all aspects of perinatal mental health. Nonetheless, within these limitations I will now attempt to discuss this topic to convey some of the skills required of the midwife. I hope this chapter will be relevant and interesting if you are considering midwifery as a career. This will apply if you are already qualified as a nurse or other professional considering a change of career, or if you are hoping to enter midwifery straight from school or college.

Pregnancy can be a time of psychological change that poses huge challenges and can cause insecurities and anxieties for the woman (Cantwell and Cox 2006). Thus, the common perception in society that being pregnant is a happy, carefree time can be quite the opposite experience for many women; this can further compound their anxieties (Muir 2007). The following excerpt is taken from my own research and is based on a real-life situation (Forrest 2004). This woman was unable to reveal her depression to her husband or her family, due to a loss of confidence in herself. She did not want to disappoint them, as she felt they had expectations of her; she therefore continued struggling to keep up the pretence of normality. In doing so she said:

My husband knew absolutely nothing about it, never knew anything about me going to the doctors. I walked about with dark glasses on constantly. You know, it's funny, but I did believe that 'right well, they can't see me if I put these on' and I really just went about as if I was invisible. 'Please don't look at me.'

The midwife can have a positive impact on the woman just by taking time to listen. Another example from my study demonstrates how another woman was able to 'open up' because the midwife showed interest in her problems:

I think initially you can tell when there is somebody there that is sympathetic, that will listen, that may say something when you walk out the door, but at least they are there, they are listening to you, you feel they look interested.

The importance of the midwife as a public health practitioner, and crucial to enhancing overall health, has been clearly shown by research (Ó Lúanaigh and Carlson 2005). Midwifery practice has always engaged public health issues, although this has not always been instantly recognisable. It is important that midwives acknowledge this important aspect of their role and continue to make a real difference to the public health of women and families. As an example of this, the midwife can provide information, advice and support on issues such as screening, testing, supplementation, for example with folic acid, stopping smoking, breastfeeding promotion and immunisation.

Although not directly mentioned here, the midwife can identify the woman with particular needs and develop services to support her. This includes mental health needs. Postnatal depression is one aspect of perinatal mental illness that is regarded as being a depressive illness occurring during the first postnatal year. The term 'perinatal mental health' relates to the emotional well-being of parents and infants in the antenatal and postnatal period up to about one year after the birth of the baby. Between 10 and 15 per cent of women suffer from postnatal depression (PND) following childbirth (O'Hara and Swain 1996). Until recently, depression arising during pregnancy was not considered; but mental ill health may commence in the antenatal period for a significant proportion of women (Andersson *et al.* 2003). Therefore, the term 'perinatal mental health' has allowed a more complete approach to be adopted, which not only considers postnatal problems such as depression, but aspects of how becoming a parent can have an impact on adult mental health. This also addresses existing mental illness and how it can impact on the ability to parent adequately and how it may affect the parent–infant attachment and subsequent relationship. Therefore, the emphasis on providing a more holistic approach to care to minimise mental health problems within the perinatal period is worth consideration (Austin 2003).

Guidance

Our practice as midwives is specifically guided by the Nursing and Midwifery Council (NMC), who produce *Midwives Rules and Standards* (NMC 2004), which must be followed. In relation to perinatal mental health, there are also:

- The recommendations made by publications such as the Scottish Intercollegiate Guidelines Network (SIGN 2002).
- More recently, the National Institute for Health and Clinical Excellence (NICE), an independent organisation responsible for providing national guidance on promoting good health and preventing and treating ill health, has provided a national clinical guideline for antenatal and postnatal mental health (2007). This guideline (45) specifically only considers the treatment of mental health problems when a pregnancy is being planned, during pregnancy and in the first year after giving birth, therefore is of particular relevance to the work of midwives.
- Additionally, the Confidential Enquiries into Maternal Deaths (CEMD), *Why Mothers Die 1997–1999* report (2001), and the Confidential Enquiry into Maternal and Child Health (CEMACH), *Why Mothers Die 2000–2002* (2004) report, gave midwives information on maternal deaths related to the childbirth period. This CEMACH report cited psychiatric illness as the most common cause of indirect deaths and the largest cause of maternal deaths overall between 1997 and 2002. More recently, however, the CEMACH *Saving Mothers' Lives* report (2007) has indicated that suicide was no longer the leading cause of indirect maternal deaths during the period 2003–2005. However, it is unclear whether this is as a result of enhanced midwifery care or due to an increase in other causes.

These reports and documents have led to the recognition that perinatal mental illness is a major issue. They also warn against the flippant use of the term PND, to the detriment of acknowledging a more serious condition. Despite this, a lot of focus is still placed on the detection and prevention of PND. The NICE clinical guideline 45 (2007) for antenatal and postnatal mental health recognises that many women have levels of depression, anxiety and distress that may not be severe enough for referral to specialist services; it is for this large group of women that midwives can play an important role in offering support. To help with this, the midwife takes a detailed history from each pregnant woman, which includes all obstetric factors and psychosocial issues. It is important for the midwife to remember that normal emotional changes at this time in a woman's life may mask depressive symptoms or be misinterpreted as depression (SIGN 2002).

The midwife's knowledge and role

To avoid or minimise problems, the midwife requires an in-depth knowledge of the risk factors for perinatal illness. To do this effectively, the midwife must also have good communication and listening skills, to be able to collect this information sensitively from the woman and build a trusting, therapeutic relationship. Although we know from the literature (NICE 2007) that detecting antenatal risk factors does not predict postnatal illness, it can alert midwives to the possibility, and encourage communication between the health care team. As suggested by NICE clinical guideline 45 (2007), each health care professional involved in the care of a childbearing woman should ask her two questions to identify possible depression at her first (booking) contact and in the postnatal period. This emphasises the multiprofessional team approach to caring for women during this time and includes the midwife, obstetrician, health visitor and GPs. The two recommended questions are:

1   During the past month, have you often been bothered by feeling down, depressed or hopeless?
2   During the past month, have you often been bothered by having little interest or pleasure in doing things?

A third question should be considered if the woman answers 'yes' to either of the initial questions:

3   Is this something you feel you need or want help with?

The midwife is ideally placed to ask these questions and to communicate with the wider multidisciplinary team. The midwife sees the woman when she attends the GP to have her pregnancy confirmed, or at her booking visit in early pregnancy. Each midwife would discuss any concerns with midwifery, obstetric, social work or mental health colleagues. In the event of needing to admit a woman and her baby for specialist care, a team approach to this decision is necessary, including the woman's family (SIGN 2002). The midwife assumes a particular role in working closely with perinatal mental health teams. Joint midwifery, obstetric and psychiatric care can be provided throughout pregnancy, with planning for the birth and postnatal care of the woman and her baby. This is an important liaison role, which forges better understanding of each team member's contribution and better working relations between different professional groups. A plan known as an 'integrated care pathway', involving midwifery, obstetric and psychiatric care, is an example of 'good practice', in which the midwife is instrumental.

The woman and her family

It is important for the midwife to involve the woman in decision making about her care. This aspect is crucial to Scotland's maternity services and is outlined in the document, A Framework for Maternity Services in Scotland (SEHD 2001). This aspect supports joint working between women, their families and the team of professionals involved in their care. This involves the midwife striving for a particular standard of care to ensure that the needs of the woman are met. This is particularly important not only for the woman, but also for her family. Research in this area has shown that perinatal mental health problems in women can result in long-term mental health difficulties for the whole family and, particularly, the children (O'Connor et al. 2002). It has also been found that the woman with perinatal mental health problems may not seek treatment. This may be due to the perceived stigma of mental health problems, as well as the woman's unrealistic expectations of motherhood (McIntosh 1993). Recent studies have shown that the detection of PND increases with routine screening. Thus, training health professionals in screening would increase awareness of perinatal mental health problems and make services more responsive to the woman's needs (Buist et al. 2006).

The woman's background

When taking a woman's history, it is important to know the nature of any past or current illness. This ensures that the best care can be provided and tailored for the individual woman's situation and involves relevant health professionals. For example, the midwife needs to know whether:

- there is any known health problem;
- the woman is currently taking medication;
- she has ever been admitted to hospital;
- if so, how long the illness lasted;
- she attends for support and to whom?

It is also important to be able to distinguish any risk factors by gaining information about any family history. The midwife would want to know such things as:

- the nature of the illness;
- that person's relationship to the childbearing woman.

In particular, a close relative with a severe condition, such as bipolar disorder or possibly schizophrenia, puts a woman at greater risk of perinatal illness. This is most likely to manifest itself as a psychotic illness, which is a serious episode of mental illness in the postnatal period. Obviously, this could have significant consequences for the woman and her family (Cantwell and Smith 2006).

The midwife should always offer the woman the opportunity to have 'private time' with her. This would allow discussion of any issues in confidence, without other family members being present. This can pose more of a problem when the community midwife is seeing a woman at home, as there are often family members around. However, the midwife frequently sees the woman at home as part of her community practice. Because of this the midwife becomes intuitive and adaptive if she suspects that there is a problem, but the woman has difficulty discussing it. The midwife would arrange another visit, when the woman would have more privacy to discuss such issues.

The need for 'private time' between the woman and professionals originated with the recognition of the high incidence of domestic abuse (WHO 1997, 2002). Despite the frequency of domestic abuse during the childbearing years (Johnson *et al.* 2003) there are still many unanswered questions regarding its precise prevalence. Similarly, risk factors for the woman, her unborn baby and the subsequent consequences of this victimisation are not clear (Jasinski 2004). I have only briefly alluded to this topic within my discussion of perinatal mental health and the role of the midwife. With increasing know-ledge, active involvement and as part of their overall public health role, the midwife asks the woman about the risk of harm at home. You may be aware that any woman affected by domestic abuse is at higher risk of developing problems such as depression; she generally lacks support, and often feels isolated. As mentioned before, it is crucial for the midwife to recognise the more vulnerable woman. This includes women living with abuse, very young women, homeless women or women from ethnic minorities, especially where there is a language barrier. Often, if social support is lacking, there may be financial and housing difficulties, which can lead to lowered mood or depression (Ó'Lúanaigh and Carlson 2005).

After the birth of the baby

The postnatal period is a busy time for the midwife, in that she has to observe both the woman and the baby. The emotional well-being of the woman, and her bonding and attachment with her baby, is just one aspect of midwifery care, as there are many physical checks that should be made. The midwife has to be aware, however, of any factors that potentially put the woman at greater risk of mental illness at this time. For example, it is not always easy to ascertain what a 'difficult birth' is. There are some associations between women who had their first baby by Caesarean, or experienced obstetric complications, and the risk of developing postnatal depression (SIGN 2002). However, the expectation of the individual woman has to be considered, and a woman may report, following what the midwife thinks is a 'normal birth', that it had been a terrible experience for her. This may be a contributing factor or cause of her depression (SIGN 2002; NICE 2007). Often her perception of how well she was supported and involved in the decision-making process will have an influence on her emotional state (SIGN 2002; NICE 2007).

It may be that women who are severely affected by the 'baby blues' are more likely to go on to develop postnatal depression (SIGN 2002). Today, the length of stay in hospital varies greatly. As a result, many women are discharged home by the time any 'blues' become evident. So the community midwife has to be particularly vigilant in her postnatal observations of the woman at home.

In the early postnatal period, the midwife should be alerted to any potential risks of severe mental illness by the woman's antenatal records. In this event, a postnatal plan of action would be in place for the midwife to implement after the woman has given birth. This would be based on the antenatal history, which would have ascertained any past history of severe conditions, such as puerperal psychosis, or other mental illness. A known family history of bipolar disorder, or if the woman had been noted to have depression in her pregnancy, would also alert the midwife.

A questionnaire that helps screening for postnatal depression is the Edinburgh Postnatal Depression Scale (EPDS) (Cox and Holden 1994). It is currently used by the health visitor to screen for depression in the postnatal period. It is the role of the midwife, however, to liaise with the GP and health visitor, who will continue care of the woman beyond the midwife's visits.

The midwife is required to visit the woman until ten days post-natally. She can, however, visit for longer if necessary (NMC 2004). The extended role of the midwife is under discussion and the benefits for the midwife and the woman remain uncertain; this is partly because such extended postnatal visiting encroaches on the role of other health professionals. The NMC (2004) is clear within its rules and standards for practice for midwives, stating that midwives must only undertake extended roles if they are sufficiently trained to do so. However, as a midwife with many years of experience working with women and families, together with teaching and research, I believe the best way forward for women is working as a team to share information effectively. This would enable a seamless service to be provided in order to meet the needs of each individual woman.

Conclusion

In this chapter I have only been able to allude to some of the aspects of perinatal mental health care that the midwife provides. This service can vary widely depending on where the midwife practises, such as in rural or urban settings. Despite this, each midwife practises with clear guidance from the NMC (2004). There is, however, much scope to develop roles and services depending on the needs of women and their families. If you have a particular interest in perinatal mental health, there are many sources within the literature, journals, textbooks, websites, local and national organisations and Government documents to widen your appreciation of this very important topic. We should always remember that a woman's perinatal mental health is of the utmost importance, not only to her own well-being, but to that of her children, partner and wider family.

Commentary

Gaining valuable training and experience in Australia, Eleanor was one of the first midwives to specialise in perinatal mental health there. Returning to Scotland, Eleanor was able to apply this experience and forge for herself a similar position there. Her chapter draws on a wealth of experience of working with women and families in this area and highlights an area of importance to women and midwives. It is a topic that has failed to attract the attention it needs for many years and this is only now beginning to be addressed. Eleanor has highlighted the need for all midwives to be aware of this issue in their everyday practice, particularly in the antenatal and postnatal periods.

Although in the UK there are still only a few midwives who specialise in this area, there is the potential to do so. Some advanced qualifications are now available to enable midwives (and other health professionals) to work with women who require special help and support in this field. It is essential that midwives take advantage of such opportunities and try to improve the statistics.

Eleanor also writes about the need for teamwork in this area, thereby capturing an essential element of midwifery practice in most settings. In the normal pregnancy continuum midwives are indeed the experts, but when dealing with acute or chronic medical or psychiatric conditions, such as postnatal depression or other mental health issues, it is vital that the midwife works with other professionals so that the woman can have a well-coordinated approach to her care and treatment.

References

Andersson, L., Sundstrom-Poromaa, I., Bixo, M. and Wulff, M. (2003) 'Point prevalence of psychiatric disorders during the second trimester of pregnancy: a population based study', *American Journal of Obstetrics & Gynecology* 189(1): 148–54.

Austin, M.-P (2003) 'Perinatal mental health: opportunities and challenges for psychiatry', *Australasian Psychiatry* 11(4): 399–402.

Buist, A., Condon, J. and Brooks, J. *et al.* (2006) 'Acceptability of routine screening for perinatal depression', *Journal of Affective Disorders* 93: 233–7.

Cantwell, R. and Cox, J. (2006) 'Psychiatric disorders in pregnancy and the puerperium', *Current Obstetrics & Gynaecology* 16: 14–20.

Cantwell, R. and Smith, S. (2006) 'Prediction and prevention of perinatal mental illness', *Psychiatry* 5(1): 15–21.

Confidential Enquiries into Maternal Deaths (CEMD) in the UK (2001) *Why Mothers Die 1997–1999*, London: RCOG Press.

Confidential Enquiry into Maternal and Child Health (CEMACH) (2004) *Why Mothers Die 2000–2002*, London: RCOG Press.

Confidential Enquiry into Maternal and Child Health (CEMACH) (2007) *Saving Mothers' Lives: Reviewing maternal deaths to make motherhood safer 2003–2005*, London: RCOG Press.

Cox, J. and Holden, J. (1994) *Perinatal Psychiatry: Use and misuse of the Edinburgh Postnatal Depression Scale*, London: Gaskell.

Forrest, E. (2004) 'A grounded theory study of services for postnatal depression: women's experiences and perceptions', unpublished M.Phil. thesis, Glasgow Caledonian University.

Jasinski, J.L. (2004) 'Pregnancy and domestic violence: a review of the literature', *Journal of Trauma, Violence & Abuse* 5(1): 47–64.

Johnson, J.K., Haider, F., Ellis, K., Hay, D.M. and Lindow, S.W. (2003) 'The prevalence of domestic violence in pregnant women', *BJOG: An International Journal of Obstetrics & Gynaecology* 110(3): 272–5.

McIntosh, J. (1993) 'Postpartum depression: women's help-seeking behaviour and perceptions of cause', *Journal of Advanced Nursing* 19: 178–84.

Muir, A. (2007) *Overcome Your Postnatal Depression*, London: Hodder Arnold.

National Institute for Health and Clinical Excellence (NICE) (2007) *Antenatal and Postnatal Mental Health: Clinical management and service guidance*, Guideline 45, London: NICE.

Nursing and Midwifery Council (NMC) (2004) *Midwives Rules and Standards*, London: NMC.

O'Connor, T., Heron, J., Golding, J., Beveridge, M. and Glover, V. (2002) 'Maternal antenatal anxiety and children's behaviour/emotional problems at 4 years', *British Journal of Psychiatry* 180: 502–8.

O'Hara, M. and Swain, A. (1996) 'Rates of postpartum depression', *International Review of Psychiatry* 8(1): 37–54.

Ó Lúanaigh, P. and Carlson, C. (2005) *Midwifery and Public Health: Future directions and new opportunities*, London: Elsevier.

Price, S. (ed.) (2007) *Mental Health in Pregnancy and Childbirth*, Edinburgh: Churchill Livingstone.

Royal College of Midwives (RCM) (2008) *Becoming a Midwife*, 21 May. Available online at www.rcm.org.uk/jobs-and-careers/becoming-a-midwife/?locale=en (accessed 3 November 2008).

Royal College of Midwives (RCM) (2008) *Working for Midwives*, 24 September. Available online at www.rcm.org.uk/college/about-us/?locale=en (accessed 3 November 2008).

Scottish Executive Health Department (SEHD) (2001) *A Framework for Maternity Services in Scotland*, Edinburgh: HMSO.

Scottish Intercollegiate Guidelines Network (SIGN) (2002) *Management of Postnatal Depression and Puerperal Psychosis*, Guideline 60, Edinburgh: SIGN Executive.

World Health Organisation (WHO) (1997) *Violence Against Women*, WHO Consultation. Available online at www.who.int/gender/violence/en/ (accessed 19 December 2008).

World Health Organisation (WHO) (2002) *World Report on Violence and Health*, WHO, Geneva. Available online at www.who.int/gender/violence/en/ (accessed 19 December 2008).

Part 2

The midwife and the wider environment

Chapter 5

The midwife manager

Georgina Sosa

Introduction

It's Sunday, my day off: my brain feels fresh and revitalised. I take advantage of this by planning the coming week and getting ready to review the staffing and budget sheets. I need to assess, once again, why the pharmacy budget is over the limit this month. At times like this, I question the connection I now have with the women I serve. A quick reflection of my management role, however, reassures me that, although some aspects of my role are indirect, they do have a major impact on the service and our working environment. This energises me to complete the tasks as, after 13 years of working as a midwife and midwife manager, I am still passionate about improving midwifery practice and the services for women. My ardent interest in midwifery, however, began years before my midwifery training . . . .

It was 1982 and I was 12 years old . . . that was when I made a conscious decision that I was going to be a midwife. First, my decision was influenced when I watched the care provided for my mother and some events at her home birth. I was privileged to witness the special connection and trust that a woman and midwife develop on their journey together. Second, my decision was influenced by two neighbours who were midwives; both had over 30 years' experience. They appeared very dedicated, kind, compassionate and positive and had high energy levels, while making time to listen and advise.

I looked up to these midwives due to their independence and professionalism. While my mother was pregnant, I felt safe knowing that these midwives lived next door and could help if necessary, as my mother was having a home birth. These midwives had a special connection within the community that they served, as they lived as part of it in a council flat in Hackney. I could not imagine a doctor living in such circumstances. Over ten years later, I started my midwifery career there.

One of the midwives was Caucasian and had retired, but still worked at the local family planning clinic. She was very funny and easygoing; the other midwife was West Indian, was more quiet and serious, and was a midwifery manager. They gave me my first insight into a profession that embraced diversity and equality of race and empowered women to progress in a profession. This was a powerful image for me as I came from a working-class, very multicultural/multiracial family and I felt very strongly about women's rights. The midwives projected that midwifery was a career in which women could excel as independent professionals. I still feel that this is the case. At such a young age, I could not tell you what the role of a policeman, teacher, priest, doctor, fireman or dentist entailed, but I could tell you the role of the midwife. I later learned that 'midwife' means 'with woman'. I already understood this concept, as I had seen and felt that meaning. What I observed as a child gave me enough ambition and inspiration to fuel my journey to becoming a midwife, and a midwife manager.

Throughout my mother's pregnancies, I attended the antenatal checks and listened to my brother's and sister's heartbeats. I observed how the midwives were advocates for my mother, trying to find a GP to attend her home birth in the early 1980s. My mother was determined and expressed that she had achieved a home birth with less resistance ten years earlier. Beech (2006) observes that changes happened in 1970 when the Peel Report (1970) stated: 'the resources of modern medicine should be available to all mothers and babies, and we think that sufficient facilities should be provided to allow for 100% hospital delivery.'

Beech (2006) argued that no one asked the mothers if they would prefer to give birth in hospital and no evidence was presented to support the claim that hospitals were safer than women's homes. The Peel Report was reinforced by the Government's Maternity Services Advisory Committee (1984), which argued that the practice of delivering nearly all babies in hospital had contributed to the dramatic reduction in baby deaths and to the avoidance of many handicaps (Osbourne 2004). This statement was made before the huge contribution of social well being to health was recognised.

I appreciate that it was midwives such as my neighbours who fought to provide midwifery-led care in an increasingly medicalised culture. My early recollections have made me want to replicate that unique connection between the woman and midwife, whether or not it is at home. Little did I know that, in 1995, this would start for me when I attended my first home birth, less than a mile from where I witnessed my mother's maternity care and my brother's birth.

Proactive management

The maternity climate is changing, with reforms under way to ensure woman-centred care, encouraging choice for women and families. The Government has devised targets to enhance a patient-led NHS that uses available resources as effectively and fairly as possible to promote health, reduce health inequalities and deliver the best and safest health care (DH 2004, 2006a, 2007a). As a midwife manager, I embrace these changes. I have the opportunity to challenge and lead the review of maternity services and assess whether women are receiving care that is sensitive and safe for their individual needs. I also assess whether they are receiving care at the most appropriate time in the most suitable environment. This includes promoting home birth when appropriate. It is a huge task and I have to be ready to welcome constant change. I can never sit back and think that my work is complete.

As a midwife manager, I must monitor the available resources and climate in which we work; therefore, I can prioritise which strategies are applicable and beneficial to the local services and develop action plans to accomplish the targets. There are targets and strategies, however, that are obligatory to all maternity units and it is vital that they are translated and resourced to initiate the project. An example of this is the European Working Time Directive (EWTD) (DH 2007b). The EWTD, from the Council of Europe, aims to protect the health and safety of workers. It lays down minimum requirements regarding working hours, rest periods, annual leave and working arrangements for night staff. August 2009 is the deadline for a 48-hour maximum working week (DH 2007b). To achieve this, the senior house officer (SHO/junior doctor) for obstetrics no longer works exclusively in maternity at night, but as part of the general hospital at night team. The implications for our unit were analysed and it was agreed to employ an extra senior midwife at night. The role of this midwife was scrutinised, as the obstetricians' expectations were that the midwife should cover the SHO's duties. After deliberation, it was acknowledged that, unlike the SHO, this midwife must refer to the obstetric registrar when women present with abnormal symptoms and/or situations. This ensures that midwives stay within their code of conduct and contract. An additional role was added, however, to assist at a Caesarean, for which training and competence were assessed.

This move has been criticised, as it appears that midwives are stepping into the medical domain, but in reality it has proved the opposite. There are now two senior midwives at night who lead the midwifery care provided. They give a sense of security and support to other midwives and each other to proactively practise normal midwifery and help to recognise abnormalities. The women also gain, as there is more midwifery experience and knowledge to promote normality; if a Caesarean is required, there is continuity of care as familiar faces will accompany the woman to her operation, making the experience less frightening. This is potentially a win-win situation, as the hours of the SHO are reduced and the maternity unit gains an extra senior midwife to support and empower women, midwives and the obstetric registrar. The review of such an initiative is continuous, thus ensuring that midwives continue to function within their sphere of practice.

The challenge of keeping up with the current targets and strategies is not easy. I need dedication, drive, motivation, enthusiasm, assertiveness, interest, empathy, bravery and loads of energy to make things happen. The amount of literature to analyse is vast and continuous so, as well as these qualities, I have to be highly computer literate. Apart from Government strategies, there are websites and publications alerting us to potential hazards, new products and new clinical practice guidelines that require action. Analytical skills are essential, because many of the publications are long and theoretically challenging. As a midwife manager, not only do I have to make sense of these publications, but I must also translate and relay them to all staff, so that they are understood and necessary changes implemented. This process has enhanced my knowledge and increased my understanding of the midwifery profession; I am now in a good position to write policies and guidelines to improve maternity services. It is a great privilege to have access to so much literature, but it can also be overwhelming and difficult to prioritise. The information gained must be shared, however, otherwise it is useless. This is because changes cannot be accomplished at management level alone; a team approach is essential.

Change

How do you create an efficient working culture that maximises safety and quality and is cost effective, without inflicting unnecessary stress on staff? I regularly have to examine how I will change a practice, which can be difficult when certain cultures are traditionally embedded. Due to my pursuit of replicating that special connection between the midwife and the woman, my first change management project as a midwife manager was to create three birthing rooms to promote normality for women labouring in a hospital environment. Evidence supports such an initiative (Newburn and Singh 2003). Although the *idea* was welcomed, there was much resistance from midwives to the practical changes. The main concern expressed was finding emergency equipment if needed, as the three rooms were stripped of technical obstetric equipment, which was replaced by beanbags, mats, TV, radio, soft lighting and birthing balls. Listening to the staff concerns made me realise that they had the ability to analyse the details and find the solutions, which ultimately made the bigger picture of utilising the birthing rooms much more effective. Staff suggested that items of obstetric equipment, such as the foetal heart monitor, intravenous poles and pumps, were stored in the corridor to ensure their accessibility. We acknowledged that this would be a suitable solution and staff realised that they should contribute and advance their ideas. Again, this was a lesson for me – that the decisions must not stay with the managers as we don't have all the solutions. The ownership of innovation must be shared, so that the midwives become advocates of the environment and practice. With the aid of the head of midwifery, community midwife manager and the practice development midwife, we have now expanded the 'Normalising Midwifery-led Care' initiative. It addresses the clinical practice of midwives and reviews how midwives can be supported to promote normality for healthy women with straightforward pregnancies/labours. It was clear that midwives had prominent fears of labours turning abnormal. The management insight does not stop there, as we are now planning to build a separate midwifery-led unit. This process takes time, as the logistics of staffing, location, equipment and clinical guidelines must be assessed. The guidelines are intensive, as they must inform midwives regarding the inclusion and exclusion criteria for admission to the midwifery-led unit. This is one of many projects of change and innovation in progress.

Organisational issues

Experience as a midwife manager has exposed me to a predominantly twenty-first-century phenomenon: dealing with the press. Sometimes, this involves a response to negative, even scandalous, reports at local or national level. You must be precise in anything you say and ensure that it does not contradict other issues that are then questioned. Women are much more aware of the public sector services and understand their rights to a safe, high quality service. When they do not receive it, or they feel it is jeopardised, they want answers from accountable managers. This is a healthy progression and for most women and families they would not have to resort to the press. Discussions can take place face-to-face with midwives, the midwifery manager or specific specialists. The maternity services are continually assessing the views of women through questionnaires, face-to-face interviews and through Maternity Service Liaison Committees (MSLCs) (DH 2006b).

The press can be utilised positively, so that they are involved in promoting, advertising and advocating new services. We utilised the press to promote the midwifery birthing rooms and later the introduction of water births with a revamped water birth room. In our era we need to advertise, promote and inform the public about services, but again this can be accomplished on a local level through the connection between midwives and women.

Regarding the budget, I must manage it efficiently. This includes assessing the staffing, stock supplies, laundry, sterilising items, stationery and equipment required. There has to be a balance to ensure sufficient resources to cover the service demands, but to result in minimal waste. Instigating the midwifery rooms and water birth initiative introduced me to locating money with the help of maternity staff to fund projects without using the maternity budget. This is when I found that one has to be imaginative and creative, as well as using intelligence to locate resources. The NHS does not have an endless pot of money, so persuasion is necessary within the hospital, community, charity organisations and outside agencies to obtain funds for important strategies. When purchasing equipment, negotiation with suppliers is needed to achieve the best price for products. A senior midwife organised a sponsored bike ride to raise funds for the equipment to help normalise birth. I had to urge caution, however, regarding the health and safety aspects – I feel at times that I put a damper on certain events. I learnt very quickly, though, that risk, accountability, liability and litigation are very much part of working in the modern NHS. At the centre of all care is the need to ensure the safety of the mother and baby. As a manager I must also ensure the safety of staff and that they are working within safe operational systems.

Risk

Risk management is a large part of my role. This includes proactive and reactive assessments to assess the probability of potentially harmful events occurring, or to assess an event that has already occurred. I investigate cases to find out why the adverse event happened and analyse what recommendations can be stipulated and disseminated in response. My role has increased in this domain to include debriefing women after they have experienced events that have left them with issues. These issues may be as a consequence of women not being able to let go, as they do not remember all the events, or do not understand and/or did not agree with the events that took place. Women are now much more aware and knowledgeable about what happens to their bodies. As midwives, we encourage and empower women to have control regarding their choices, especially when they feel vulnerable. Some women are anxious in their current pregnancy due to their previous experience of labour and delivery. Through debriefing, I listen to and acknowledge the woman's experience, using her maternity records to portray the midwives' and obstetricians' documentation. I have learnt that honesty with the woman and using her maternity records are the best tools for the woman to reflect, understand and start to make sense of the events and work towards closure. The aspect of honesty includes apologising and acknowledging when we got it wrong for a woman. This is a scary concept when litigation is prominent in maternity, but sometimes that is what is needed . . . an apology. Following such circumstances, it is my role to formulate a review of the organisational systems and/or clinical practices to ensure that lessons are learnt and a proactive stance is taken to prevent the episode recurring. Occasionally, the review will involve assessing the clinical practice of an individual or individuals, whether it is an obstetrician, anaesthetist, midwife or midwifery support worker. I have to ensure that this is instigated by the appropriate person and provide feedback. This is also a new concept of midwives questioning the practice of doctors. As one of the leaders in the maternity services, I have to push the boundaries as much as is safely possible to avoid inter- ventions such as unnecessary Caesareans and their associated risk factors (Mander 2007). If this process is not completed, a woman loses confidence in the maternity services and cannot feel safe, which means that she will find it difficult to experience a trusting connection with the midwife.

All midwives are autonomous practitioners, but as a midwife manager I am responsible for the organisational systems within which they work. I work with the practice development midwife to make certain that appropriate training is available and that staff attend. In addition, I must ensure that there are efficient systems in place to monitor the practice of maternity staff. The training and monitoring prepares them to work at their full potential while remaining within their sphere of practice, with the correct skills and at the appropriate level to provide safe, quality maternity care. At the same time, I must try to ensure that staff do not become demoralised from aspiring to unrealistic standards. If staff are demoralised they risk losing the human connection that midwives have with women, which is as important to women as midwives' intellect and clinical practice.

Crisis

This involves the unexpected or the foresight of a potential problem evolving that could have significant consequences. I have to think on my feet and react quickly with a plan of action. Some incidents can be very serious, with catastrophic consequences. In such circumstances, the situation must be immediately investigated and the plan of management must involve the inclusion of the appropriate people to assess and help resolve the situation. We are a 24/7 service, so the crisis can occur at any time. The organisational systems are crucial in these incidents, so that midwives know how to manage the situation safely and know who to contact for clinical and/or managerial support. The women and families must be kept informed at all times, especially when the health of the woman and/or baby has been at risk, requiring emergency treatment. Again, from experience, the woman gains trust and respect for the midwives if she understands the journey that resulted in the unexpected events.

Having worked as a midwife in London, I learned the reasons why there were not enough staff, that is, short-term and long-term sickness, maternity leave, study leave and particular problems around holiday periods. This was particularly difficult when activity was high on the labour ward. I was familiar with calling in extra staff and prioritising the work, in order to ensure that the care provided was safe while trying to avoid the maternity unit closing, as this meant the women would have to travel to the nearest labour ward until beds and/or staff were available. On moving to Norfolk five years ago, I encountered another unforeseen situation that can affect the efficiency of the workforce: a severe weather warning. This can have a major impact on the staffing levels and skill mix of staff. I did not just have to worry about myself getting into work, but the whole workforce. When I was faced with such an unexpected challenge, I realised that I did have the knowledge to juggle staff shifts, but it required teamwork, as flexibility and goodwill from all the maternity staff were crucial. I quickly realised that the women would also experience problems getting to the hospital. Contingency plans with the community management, midwives and ambulance crews had to be prepared to advise women appropriately. I now find myself keeping a watchful eye on the weather forecast. Having the foresight to anticipate predicaments is vital. This is something we discovered when large numbers of midwives were going off on maternity leave at the same time, which was definitely going to have an impact on midwifery staffing and the skill mix. This emphasises that the midwife manager needs to see the bigger picture and realise the solutions while empowering the team to accomplish it.

The personal aspects of being a midwifery manager

I did not set out to be a midwifery manager, but I fell into the role as a natural progression. This does not mean that the position fell into my lap, however, as selection was a competitive and intellectually challenging process. I originally intended to be the best midwife that I could be and progress academically, just as many of my experienced colleagues have. I specialised as a female genital mutilation midwife, and achieved a first-class honours degree and M.Sc. while working as a midwife in North London. The academic experience developed my political astuteness, but I have known midwives who have acquired such skills with years of experience. When I moved to Norfolk, I took a job as a senior midwife on a labour ward, which was the equivalent to my position in London. When a labour ward manager position was advertised, I realised that my experience in London equipped me for it. The management experience gave me insight to progress to the position of clinical midwifery manager for hospital services. Experience is a vital commodity for management; as I have said, you need insight and to be able to see the bigger picture, so that you can lead the services. When I was a junior midwife in North London I was surrounded every day by midwives with 20–30 years' midwifery experience. I felt so safe and nurtured in their presence and it was as though they were passing a baton of experience over to me to pass on to the next generation of midwives. In Norfolk, the head of midwifery and clinical midwifery manager for community services now act as my management mentors. They, with other midwives with years of experience, still enhance my midwifery practice. Every midwife needs inspiration to carry on, as occasionally morale falters, whether it is due to a sad, difficult clinical event, overwhelming workload or shortages of resources. Initially, I passed my baton to student midwives; but then the spectrum broadened as my experience extended and, like so many generations of midwives before me, I now teach obstetricians too.

The responsibility as a midwife manager is difficult to communicate; but my family understand it by the excessive hours I work, as it is not unusual that I return home late, or miss special family and social events, due mostly to unexpected crises at work. When I am at home my mind is easily distracted by thinking about work. I am fortunate to have a very understanding family, in particular my husband, who has witnessed my journey and passion for midwifery. I can now understand why my neighbour, who was the district midwifery manager, was more reserved and serious; she was probably distracted by work innovations and demands. These themes are familiar to many managers and, through experience, a better work–life balance can be achieved through different working arrangements.

Not all midwifery managers' positions are the same. The beauty is that each maternity unit can individualise the role to suit its culture and dynamics. My position has progressed to three days management and two days clinical, because we are a small maternity unit. This gives me time to assess and deliver the leadership and management responsibilities, but, at the same time, not lose my clinical skills or contact with women and staff. I therefore keep an awareness of midwifery practice, which is crucial

The pinnacle for me is still that special connection between the woman and me; this is particularly felt at the point just before the birth, when both mother and midwife put so much faith and trust in each other's capabilities, just like that experienced by my mother and her midwives.

Now, where are those budget sheets?. . .

Commentary

Georgina's account of what she does as a midwife manager brings to life a neglected area of midwifery. We are shown clearly the highs and lows of the manager's role.

Particularly important in Georgina's narrative is her emphasis on what she calls 'the bigger picture'. All too often the focus is on the minutiae and the details of micro-management. For the manager to be able to contextualise her work is admirable and appears to be satisfying.

Another interesting issue arising from Georgina's chapter is found in her frequent mention of 'serving' and 'service'. This is an aspect of midwifery, and health care generally, which has largely been forgotten or ignored with increasing professionalisation. Occasionally, as Mary Cronk (2005) has done, we need to be reminded of the focus of midwifery and the relationship between the midwife and childbearing woman.

This relationship is described by Georgina as 'connection' and underpins all that the midwife does. Others have used the term 'partnership' to indicate this crucial relationship and words such as engagement and empathy also feature.

Georgina shows the importance of her personal experience of her family background and gives credit to her husband for his forbearance. Interestingly, though, she does not raise her personal childbearing experience, the significance of which is discussed in Chapter 14.

References

Beech, B. (2006) 'At last: an NMC home birth circular', *AIMS Journal* 18(1). Available online at www.aims.org.uk/Journal/Vol18No1/NMC HomebirthCircular.htm (accessed 29 April 2008).

Cronk, M. (2005) 'Guest editorial. Midwives: professional servants?', *RCM Midwives* 8(6): 240.

Department of Health (DH) (1970) *The Peel Report*, London: HMSO.

Department of Health (DH) (2004) *National Service Framework for Children, Young People and Maternity Services*, published 14 September, London: DH.

Department of Health (DH) (2006a) *Health Reform in England: Update and commissioning framework*, published 13 July, London: DH.

Department of Health (DH) (2006b) *National Guidelines for Maternity Services Liaison Committees (MSLCs)*, published 13 February, London: DH. Available online at www.dh.gov.uk/en/publicationsandstatistics/publications/publicationspolicyandguidance/dh_4128339 (accessed 30 August 2008).

Department of Health (DH) (2007a) *Maternity Matters: Choice, access and continuity of care in a safe service*, London: DH.

Department of Health (DH) (2007b) *What is the European Working Time Directive?* London: DH, last modified 9 August. Available online at www.dh.gov.uk/en/Managingyourorganisation/Humanresourcesandtraining/Modernisingworkforceplanninghome/Europeanworkingtimedirective/index.htm (accessed 30 August 2008).

Mander, R. (2007) *Caesarean: Just another way of birth?* London: Routledge.

Maternity Services Advisory Committee (1984) *Report to the Secretaries of State for Social Services and for Wales, Part II: Care during childbirth*, London: HMSO.

Newburn, M. and Singh, D. (2003) *Creating a Better Birth Environment Report: Women's views about the design and facilities in the maternity units – a national survey*. London: The National Childbirth Trust. Available online at www.nctpregnancyandbabycare.com/about-us/what-we-do/campaigning/better-birth-environment (accessed 12 November 2008).

Osbourne, A. (2004) 'A culture of fear: the midwifery perspective', *Midwifery Matters* 100, Spring, Association of Radical Midwives, London. Available online at www.radmid.demon.co.uk/A%20Culture%20of%20Fear.htm (accessed 29 April 2008).

Chapter 6

The midwife who is in education

Elma Paxton

When deciding to become a midwife many years ago, I little realised the opportunities it could provide. I knew of the skills I would gain and the potential to work abroad was also an exciting possibility. However, I little realised the direction that my career would take, leading me to continue my own education at university, via teaching certificates and a bachelor's degree to a master's degree. In the near future, I will retire from a career in midwifery that has spanned almost 40 years, and that has allowed me to work in many settings in several countries. I will finish my working life as a university lecturer, a position of which I never dreamt when I set out to become a midwife.

When midwifery students arrive at university for the first day of orientation, each person has a unique story. Interest in midwifery as a profession will have been stimulated in different ways. For some, it will be the next step following secondary education; for others it will be a career change. University life holds many challenges and balancing academic, professional and personal demands can be onerous. As adult learners the motivation is personal and tangible, but on the pathway the midwife in education will facilitate the individual and nurture teamwork.

The focus of this chapter is the student experience through the eyes of both educator and student. For this reason, the contribution, enthusiasm and ongoing commitment of students to midwifery as a profession are acknowledged. The midwife who is an educator has the inherent belief that sees in her students the capacity to lead and to enlarge midwifery. This chapter builds on the experiences portrayed by students in the introductory chapter.

Background

Historically, the recognition that midwifery is a profession distinct from other health care professions has been hard won. The struggle for autonomy and the development of a midwifery curriculum have been essential to the growth of the profession (Fleming 2002; Baird 2007). Midwifery knowledge and practice are rooted in the woman's and her family's experience of childbirth. Midwifery philosophy recognises not only a difference in the boundaries of practice, but also in the essence of practice between midwifery and other health professions. To subordinate midwifery to the medical profession (Mander and Fleming 2002) contracts the profession, to the detriment of women. The art and science of midwifery hold a unique body of knowledge, which can essentially reduce the level of medical intervention, and can give women a more fulfilling experience of childbirth. The level of awareness students have of this may vary when they first enter the university, depending on their life experiences.

Midwifery education in the UK is a marriage of apprenticeship to higher education, with a minimum of 50 per cent of the student experience being gained in practice. Apprenticeship systems were common across Europe from the early sixteenth century (Bakos 1999) and continue today. Many European countries are reluctant to give up the apprenticeship system of training, seeing in it the fundamental model for 'being with women', which defines midwifery. The disadvantage of such a system, however, lies in the perpetuation of traditional practices that are unquestioned. Some practices are rich and beneficial, while others would not stand the scrutiny of current evidence for best practice. The midwife who is in education has the opportunity to facilitate students in evaluating evidence to inform practice. The modern student is in a position to challenge practice, if it is not evidence based and of a high standard. Midwives in clinical practice similarly mentor students in a way that integrates theory and practice, and work closely with educators to ensure the best practice-based experience. The mentor is a role model for students, and will hold together education and experience, having undergone educational preparation for mentorship (NMC 2008).

The midwifery educator in higher education

The midwifery educator has a dual role, bringing together the professions of midwifery and teaching. This duality of practice needs to be held as a single entity in order to be student centred in approach to learning, and woman centred in approach to practice. When a midwife begins on the path to becoming a university lecturer, she or he will already hold a degree, and have extensive practice knowledge. Those studying to become midwifery educators will work towards a postgraduate certificate or diploma in education, which is also recognised by the NMC. During the programme, the educator will explore student learning styles and approaches to adult learning. While also giving lectures, her or his role will be to facilitate student learning, and students will be active in the learning process. This is very different from the traditional lecturer role, where students were considered passive recipients of knowledge.

The midwifery educator will be involved with students in many exciting projects throughout a programme of active learning in university and practice settings. Before entry to a midwifery programme, prospective students will already have begun active preparation in order to ensure that their educational background and life experience give them an advantage in the selection process.

The midwife as an admissions tutor

The admissions tutor may have prolonged contact with prospective students before they begin a programme of study. The tutor has a wide network of contacts in secondary and further education, liaising with schools and college careers advisers. He or she will participate in schools and university open days, take informal inquiries, review applications and participate at each stage of the selection process. This role is vital to the success of programmes, if candidates are to be adequately prepared and enabled to stay the course. The admissions tutor is also a good contact for women and men who have aspirations to be midwives, but have not the educational background to meet the entry criteria. The tutor can offer guidance on further education programmes that are designed to give access to higher education.

The admissions tutor is often the first point of contact to clarify the demands of a programme and to explain the commitment needed and the workload involved. Being a midwifery student entails intensive study and long hours of midwifery practice. From the first placement, students work alongside mentors who follow shift patterns. While the student is supernumerary, she or he will gain the greatest continuity of support for learning in practice by working as closely as possible to the mentor's shift. Unsocial working hours may be part of student life. It is also likely that the admissions tutor is involved in induction and orientation programmes at the beginning of the course. Prospective students may make contact with the admissions tutor as early as two years in advance of embarking on a midwifery programme, seeking careers advice and developing relevant skills and experience. Each of their stories, as they have shown you in the Introduction, is unique.

Student-centred education

Educators aim to balance the utility required by NHS employers with an educational philosophy that has an intrinsic purpose to develop the individual in unique and challenging ways. The midwife who is an educator recognises that students are on a pathway towards a professional career that will require self-regulation and self-education (NMC 2008). Midwifery competency, once achieved, requires lifelong commitment to sustain and develop. To be a safe practitioner, the midwife needs to have a reasonable degree of self-sufficiency and to utilise up-to-date knowledge in practice (Butler *et al.* 2008). Students therefore require control of their learning from the outset, even when working towards curriculum goals and outcomes. This can be fostered in several ways, such as inquiry-based learning, student seminars, projects and assignments.

Inquiry-based learning

Midwifery education programmes are more commonly founded on inquiry-based learning (IBL) or problem-based learning (PBL) approaches to education. There is no great difference between the terms, except that midwives often prefer to use the word 'inquiry' as 'problem' might suggest that something is wrong, when considering a normal life experience. IBL can bring a mixed response from students, especially if they have experience of more directed teaching:

I thought when entering the course that it was a partly medical-based subject and more would have been taught directly to us. Therefore I wish that I had been more prepared for this; I think it would have made it easier for me especially in 1st year!

(Third-year student)

A midwife undertaking a post-qualifying module in complex care midwifery by distance learning offered the following positive response to a trigger, which demonstrates enjoyment and preference for IBL:

During the midwifery school I really hated the whole issue around diabetes ... but reading for this scenario I am positively surprised how interesting it is. I like it ... what a surprise!

(Distance learner)

From the outset, IBL encourages teamwork. Students respond to triggers or scenarios typical of real-life situations that will be encountered in practice. There are several stages in working through a trigger, and students will be guided by the model used at the university. Each member will take turns at chairing the group, or acting as scribe, and the tutor will be available as a resource at the first session, and at the feedback session. The tutor is a facilitator, and his or her role is mainly to ensure that the trigger or scenario will elicit questions and responses necessary to meet the expected outcomes for the module. The tutor may respond to student requests for guidance, or on occasions prompt if an important factor is being missed. The tutor, however, does not want to upset group dynamics by taking an active role, being keen to see the group increase in confidence and self reliance.

To encourage deep learning, all students answer each question set by the group, provide feedback and debate issues, before contributions are finally collated by the scribe. Students could potentially divide up questions, but this is discouraged, as it is likely to lead to superficial knowledge in some aspects of the scenario. All IBL or PBL programmes will require students to access a range of resources, including databases, journals, books, internet, clinical guidelines and colleagues (Meddings and Porter 2008). Lectures are provided, but they are fewer than in traditional programmes and are considered as resources. There is a high level of accountability to the peer group, which evaluates the contribution of its members. IBL additionally requires students to appraise the quality of information they are inputting, so that student-led sessions are based on best evidence, and form part of student assessment.

The reflective practitioner

Students are encouraged to be reflective practitioners and will keep reflective accounts of their learning as part of their portfolios. The reflective practitioner has a deeper capacity for self-awareness, and will question and evaluate practice based on how it affects others and on the available evidence. By reflecting, students change and develop.

A key to the effectiveness of woman-centred care and student-centred education continues to be good tripartite relations between the student, the midwife educator and the mentor. The following reflective account demonstrates the significant influence the mentor can have as a good role model who can build student confidence (Jordan 2008). In this instance, the mentor was functioning as an autonomous practitioner who used her professional knowledge, skill and judgement to achieve an excellent outcome for her client and was a good person to emulate. Other midwives might have allowed doctors to make decisions and have been inappropriate role models (Bluff and Holloway 2008). To be a good partner and support for a woman in labour, a sensitive midwife responds to her as an individual.

Lorayne reflects on her experience in a midwifery-led unit, supporting Holly (not her real name), who was scared because her baby was 'the wrong way round'. (In obstetric terms, this is called an occipito-posterior position or OP for short.) As Lorayne acknowledges, the reflective practitioner speculates on how a situation might have been handled differently with further knowledge and hindsight. The following is a beautiful extract from her account, which provides some insight into the privilege of being with a woman through the birthing experience:

Holly was upset to hear that her baby was in the OP position as she had read about it and believed (as I did) that she would probably have a longer and harder labour. She also said that she was scared because her friend had an emergency Caesarean section recently, because her baby was the 'the wrong way round' too. My mentor explained to Holly that lying semi-recumbent in bed was not the best place for her to be to speed up her labour, with the baby lying in this position. If she felt up to it she should try changing to a more upright position or even use the chair and ball equipment. Holly, although upset and scared, agreed to try an upright position and move on to the equipment. Harry, her partner, was able to sit behind her and offer her support and help while using the equipment. Although Holly was tired and fed-up she explained that she would do anything to ensure that she managed a natural delivery.

At 12.00 hours Holly's contractions had become stronger since moving on to the chair and ball equipment. My mentor's instincts were right and Holly's labour was progressing well. Holly's contractions became stronger and more coordinated. She was now also using Entonox (gas and air) for pain relief and had withdrawn into herself – not wanting to 'chat' as much. Just over an hour later Holly showed signs of transition – she began to have an involuntary urge to push with almost every contraction and requested to move back to the bed. Holly remained upright, kneeling and leaning over the back of the bed. Holly managed to stay in this position for around ten minutes then turned around and sat upright in bed. At 13.25 the baby's head (vertex) was visible; at this point it was clear that Holly was pleased and a little surprised with her ability to deliver her baby. At 13.27 she gave birth to a healthy baby girl.

Lorayne entered a shortened midwifery programme of 18 months' duration, as she was a qualified nurse. The philosophy of nursing is different from that of midwifery. Evaluating the situation, Lorayne continues:

The best part of this experience was how pleased I felt for Holly. I felt so happy for her; Holly had done everything possible to ensure she delivered her baby naturally – she had come with her own hopes and fears about labour and childbirth; she was willing to work with the midwife and trust her in helping her to achieve the birth she had imagined. I was also encouraged to see that even with an OP position the midwife used her skills and knowledge to instil Holly with a sense of confidence in her body's ability to birth her baby.

The only thing I can think that was bad about this experience is that I feel I have let some women down in the past by my conformity to unit practice and by being unknowledgeable about the benefits of mobility and upright positions in labour. In my limited experience so far, when a woman is informed that her baby is in an OP position, she is offered and advised that she should consider a good form of pain relief (for example, an epidural), as her labour is likely to be long, painful and she may end up requiring some form of assistance to give birth. Pretty much a negative view of childbirth, which can only reduce a woman's confidence in her body.

I have come to realise that I'm sometimes afraid of offending women – wishing them to be as pain free and as comfortable as possible (lying back in bed). I think that this stems from my nursing as one of the main aims of nursing is to reduce suffering and pain – any patient found to be in pain would normally be seen as a poor reflection of my nursing care. This placement has helped me understand the well-being model of midwifery care better – women are in pain not because they are ill or sick (as in nursing) but because they are experiencing one of the most natural events in life – childbirth; no matter how you word it, labour is painful but it has a purpose, which for the majority is a positive one; the birth of a healthy baby!

(Lorayne Telfer 2008)

Lorayne's experience is not uncommon, and many midwives have questioned the profession's ability to maintain the unique aspects of midwifery in a culture where intervention prevails (Jordan 2008).

The elective placement

Often, the midwife who is in education appears to take a secondary role in the student experience, but is required to be at their most alert in safeguarding students and clients alike. This is particularly true of the elective placement, in which students plan and negotiate their own placement. Many university courses include this option in their programmes for those working in health disciplines. The placement is student initiated, student directed and, once the experience is completed, student evaluated, an aim being to encourage independent lifelong learning skills. It is a very fulfilling experience, but one that is not without frustrations, as much planning can go into a placement that, for some reason, does not materialise. This may be for financial reasons, particularly if the placement involves travel and accommodation, or reasons of safety in countries where there is political unrest, war or disease. Part of the planning can involve seeking funding. In this respect, the tutor can offer guidance. Funding organisations set criteria and an experienced teacher recognises 'no go' situations before too much effort goes into them.

There are generally three types of electives that students opt for: the first is consolidation of existing experience; the second is to select a model of experience that has not been offered within local NHS services; and the third is an overseas placement.

Many students choose to consolidate experience in an area of practice they have particularly enjoyed, or one in which they feel less confident, for example in caring for high-risk women. The elective placement tends to be close to the end of a programme and many students like to spend the time with a mentor who has been instrumental in their professional development earlier in the programme.

Desire to experience an alternative model of midwifery also drives student choices, and for this students negotiate with a service provider in another health board or local health authority area. Preferred placements include those that afford the potential opportunity for home birth, water birth, or experience in a free-standing birthing centre. Occasionally, a student will have the opportunity to spend an elective placement with an independent midwife.

A few students elect to undertake a placement overseas. This is probably the most challenging choice of all, particularly for those who go to a developing country. Health and safety issues need to be considered, particularly if there is rampant disease, political unrest or instability, warfare or poverty. A careful risk assessment should be undertaken and also adequate health insurance arranged. Travel might also be difficult and less safe than at home. Rewards are immense and life-changing, however, and it is always a choice to consider if personal circumstances permit. Such a placement takes longer to organise and should probably begin a year in advance.

Rhona's story

I have chosen to carry out my elective placement by returning to Nepal, to the unique culture where I once lived and gave birth to my daughter, to tell the stories and demonstrate the amazing resilience of the local women. I realised at the time that my experience as a 'westerner' of antenatal care and giving birth in Kathmandu was potentially very different [from that of] the Nepali women who I spoke with and assisted during childbirth, within an over-medicalised, outdated system. I witnessed traumatic, sometimes dangerous, practice in the hospitals and, with over 80 per cent of births taking place in the home, most without trained support, I want to find out more about these women's experiences. I had a UK system I could compare it with, I had access to 'birth literature', I could afford to pay for the services, I lived near a medical facility and I was empowered to be vocal about my personal expectations. I learnt a great deal about Nepali traditions in childbearing and was very fortunate in participating in a unique rite of passage, which included many traditional practices and rituals. I knew then there was a story to be told and exposed. I would like to fulfil a lifelong ambition to make short documentary films and complement this with my passion for midwifery and interest in women's rights and so plan to make a film while I am there. I would like to enable the empowerment of women through recording their stories of their experiences of childbirth.

I want to look at maternity services and the Nepal Government Maternity Incentive Scheme, which pays women to encourage them to attend hospital for birth. I will look at the traditional practices of childbearing and investigate the views of TBAs [traditional birth attendants] and midwives.

Professionally speaking, sharing experiences always puts into a wider context what we do and how we can do it better, undoubtedly enhancing practice and the care women receive.

Personally speaking, I am a single parent to my seven-year-old daughter and I want to show her what you can achieve in life if you take chances and try hard enough. It would be an ambition fulfilled and a dream come true to be able to do this. I have many ideas I would like to realise in film and share with people and this I see as a very good beginning.

Designing a curriculum

Many of the stories would not be written without a curriculum that allows students the opportunity to practise in a range of situations. While programmes are designed to ensure knowledgeable practitioners with essential competencies (Butler *et al.* 2008) and lifelong learning skills, a curriculum needs to be much more if it is to cultivate midwives who will make a difference to women's lives. To remain current, the midwifery curriculum is reviewed at least every five years by a review committee, which consists of university academics and resource personnel, midwifery educators, clinical midwives, students and consumer representatives. The nature of the programme will be influenced by the regional organisation of maternity services, as programme innovations are influenced by practice innovations.

Larger urban maternity services may be able to offer a specialised service not available in other areas, to meet the needs of vulnerable women. Remote and rural maternity services are likely to include a birthing service that is midwifery led.

Perinatal mental health has not received the due consideration given to the physical health and well-being of women during pregnancy, labour and postpartum. The midwife educator can make a significant contribution to redressing this. Perinatal mental health considerations are included in pre-registration programmes; however, curriculum innovation in perinatal mental health forms part of continuing professional development.

e-Learning and distance education

Like the midwife in clinical practice who enjoys her role 'being with women', the midwife educator probably gains most satisfaction in getting alongside students and seeing fulfilment in the students' personal and professional development. For this reason, e-learning presents a challenge to both the educator and the student. Distance learners are rarely, if ever, in the university building. The personal dimension can be lost if that extra level of commitment is not put into relationships. A key feature of e-learning is decentralised and open communication (Weller 2007). The success of e-learning in midwifery programmes is largely dependent on the common culture of the participants, who build an international midwifery identity, and who recognise their distinctiveness from other health professionals. Within e-learning there is a strong extracurricular element, and opportunities to build networks that extend beyond modules and programmes. The midwife as an educator facilitates this atmosphere and recognises her or his own role as a learner from other midwifery cultures. Other countries have achieved in areas where the midwife from Britain is still striving. This is particularly true when considering independent midwifery practice or freestanding birthing centres. Midwives from continental Europe, however, often identify the mechanisms that we take for granted in ensuring quality and standards of midwifery education and practice.

The dynamic of online programmes is in the discussion forums and live links achieved on a global scale. Pre-registration students frequently use an internet medium, such as Blackboard, to maintain links with the university while out in practice. The midwifery educator involved in international education can facilitate 'live links' between students and overseas midwives, setting up both formal and informal links that promote healthy international dialogue.

The future of midwifery education

In everyday practice, the midwife who is in education is engaged in the academic life of the university and also maintains links with practice. Challenges to practice credibility always confront the midwife in education. Although he or she is generally very research minded and knowledgeable about best practice, opportunities for clinical practice vary. Some have addressed this through combining the role of educator with that of researcher, or lecturer practitioner, and some through case holding. New innovative programmes also involve the student in caseload holding (Lewis *et al.* 2008a), which has been upheld as a best practice model (Lewis *et al.* 2008b)

Students have the privilege of knowing their clients throughout pregnancy and the women of seeing students develop as practitioners. The continuity experienced by women through the pregnancy continuum, birth and motherhood is rewarding for individual women and for students alike. The experience is a shared journey (Rolls and McGuinness 2007). Women have a sense of being in control of the birth experience and students likewise build confidence in independent decision making, through personally planning, delivering and evaluating a programme of care under the supervision of an experienced midwife. Students' case holding in such programmes is a joint venture between education and practice, and requires the cooperation of educators and practitioners alike. This remains futuristic for many schools of midwifery. Students, meantime, are effective participants in a range of practices that aim to be woman centred, and are encouraged to challenge practices that fall short of the ideal.

Conclusion

While midwives working in clinical areas have the privilege of hearing mothers' birth stories, the midwife who is an educator in university settings has the privilege of hearing students' stories. Some have come to the profession as second-generation midwives, where a parent has also been a midwife. To hear that a mother is still working, and of the continued enthusiasm of a daughter, is rewarding:

I came into midwifery because my Mum is a midwife, and though she is officially retired at the age of 65 this year, as she loves it so much she cannot give up completely and is almost working full-time hours on the bank. I hope it is 'in the blood' and I can follow in her footsteps.

Many students are impatient to graduate and practice full-time. The nature and quality of the care they provide is dependent on the education they receive today. While midwifery still needs to forge ahead and overcome barriers to autonomous practice, the voice of the student is more articulate through the experience of current education programmes, which will in turn influence future practice. Some examples of innovation have been explored, and many more await the prospective midwife of the future who is inspired by generations of the past (Worth 2007).

Commentary

In her time spent in midwifery education, Elma has seen and indeed initiated many changes. These changes are, for the most part, included in this chapter, which paints an exciting picture of the vast array of possibilities currently open to midwife educators. Indeed, Elma has demonstrated the concept of lifelong learning and shown how the midwife educator can contribute to this.

Elma has brought in various comments from midwifery students to illustrate her points. Readers should note that some of these are distance learners, often from countries other than that in which the educator is based, and others are home students. Indeed, web-based learning has opened up many new possibilities for midwifery education. One of the most exciting of these is the ability to educate to degree level, in another country, qualified midwives practising in countries with no university education, thus offering the opportunity for further advancement.

Elma also highlights the role of the midwife educator in curriculum development. Such a skill is vital to ensure the best possible start to a new career for students. She mentions innovative teaching and learning methods, all of which the midwife educator can develop and incorporate into a good curriculum. Students are then able to incorporate what they have learned into their practice with much more ease than if they had simply had to listen to lectures, thus reducing the theory–practice gap.

References

Baird, K. (2007) 'Exploring autonomy in education: preparing student midwives', *British Journal of Midwifery* 15(7), July: 400–5.

Bakos, A.E. (1999) ' "A knowledge speculative and practical": the dilemma of midwives' education in early modern Europe', in Whitehead, B.J. (ed.) *Women's Education in Early Modern Europe: A history 1500–1800*, London: Routledge.

Bluff, R. and Holloway, I. (2008) 'The efficacy of midwifery role models', *Midwifery* 24(3), September: 301–9.

Butler, M.M., Fraser, D.M. and Murphy, R.J.L. (2008) 'What are the essential competencies required of a midwife at the point of registration?' *Midwifery* 24(3), September: 260–9.

Fleming, V. (2002) 'Statutory control', in Mander, R. and Fleming, V. (eds) *Failure to Progress: The contraction of the midwifery profession*, London: Routledge.

Jordan, R. (2008) 'The confidence to practice midwifery: preceptor influence on student self-efficacy', *Journal of Midwifery & Women's Health* 53(5), September/October: 413–20.

Lewis, P., Fry J. and Rawnson, S. (2008a) 'Student midwife caseloading: a new approach to midwifery education', *British Journal of Midwifery* 16(8), August: 499–502.

Lewis, P., Fry J. and Rawnson, S. (2008b) 'Student midwife caseloading: embedding the concept within education' *British Journal of Midwifery* 16(10), October: 636–41.

Mander, R. and Fleming, V. (2002) *Failure to Progress: The contraction of the midwifery profession*, London: Routledge.

Meddings, F. and Porter, J. (2008) 'Selecting students for midwifery education: is PBL the answer?' *British Journal of Midwifery* 16(2), February: 84–7.

Nursing and Midwifery Council (NMC) (2008) Website: www.nmc-uk.org/.

Rolls, C. and McGuinness, B. (2007) 'Women's experiences of a follow through journey program with Bachelor of Midwifery students', *Women and Birth* 20: 149–52.

Weller, M. (2007) 'The distance from isolation. Why communities are the logical conclusion in e-learning', *Computers & Education* 49: 148–59.

Worth, J. (2007) *Call the Midwife: A True Story of the East End in the 1950s*, London: Weidenfeld & Nicolson.

Chapter 7

The supervisor of midwives

Jean Duerden

The term 'supervisor' conjures up all sorts of images. It reminds me of a foreman in a factory wearing a brown overall and supervising all the activity in his department, watching carefully for mistakes or errors in the processes and ensuring that a perfect product emerges at the end of the conveyor belt. In some ways, I suppose this could be quite a good analogy for midwifery; the supervisor of midwives (SOM) watching carefully, seeing that no mistakes are made and that only the highest standard of midwifery care is offered in the department and ensuring that the end result is the birth of a healthy baby with no ill effects on the mother. This does, however, sound somewhat inspectoral; sadly, some midwives might see supervision in that light, rather than in the supportive sense that it should be perceived. I hope to change any perception of punitive supervision to one of supportive supervision during this chapter.

As described elsewhere, just like when you tell someone you are a midwife and the person you are addressing wants to share their birth experience, the same can happen with supervision. If you tell a midwife from another hospital that you are an SOM, they will probably want to share their experience of supervision. I suppose it is only human nature that they are more likely to want to share their story if it was a particularly difficult experience and badly handled. We sometimes forget the good things that happen to us. Support from an SOM can be quite discreet and so much a part of everyday midwifery that it doesn't always provide a significant memory when having a conversation. It appears that our minds are tuned to recalling negative rather than positive events. It's a bit like newspapers only printing the bad news.

Rather than looking at the everyday type of supervision, let's instead look at an incident in a maternity unit and how it was successfully managed through supervision.

That night the maternity unit was extremely busy. It was impossible to give one-on-one care to every woman in labour. Jen, a newly qualified midwife, was caring for two women. It seemed that one of the women she was caring for, Amy, was a long way off giving birth, so she tried to focus her attention on Lizzie, whose birth appeared more imminent. Jen checked that Amy was comfortable and that her partner, Andy, was OK. Unfortunately, the CTG (cardiotocograph) trace in Lizzie's room showed signs of foetal distress, so Jen called the Registrar and Lizzie was rapidly taken to theatre for Caesarean section.

It was over an hour before Jen got back to Amy and Andy's room, where Amy was now in advanced labour. They were both very anxious as no one had been in to see them. Because no one had been observing Amy, there were no records of maternal observation and no record of the foetal monitoring or contractions, as there was no paper left in the CTG monitor; it had run out during Jen's absence. Jen realised with horror that she had not briefed the Labour Ward Coordinator when she was leaving the ward, or told her that Amy would need regular checking. Although she should have been supernumerary, the busyness of the labour ward that night had meant that the Coordinator was also caring for women in labour.

After Jen's return, Amy progressed to giving birth to a normal healthy baby, but Jen knew she had not ensured that Amy had received continuing care during her labour and what might have been haunted her and caused concern for the Labour Ward Coordinator.

Many midwives will be able to relate to this type of situation, where on some occasions the labour ward gets so busy that knowing where to prioritise care is difficult and unintentional mistakes are made. Making a mistake is punishment enough for any midwife, so the SOM realises that taking punitive action is neither fair nor appropriate. So let's see how this situation was handled by Sue, the SOM.

Sue learned about the incident when Jen phoned her soon after-wards. Jen hoped that, by contacting Sue as soon as possible after the incident, she would get the support she anticipated, which she did.

Sue knew that the outcome of this incident could have been very different and, in her long experience as an SOM, she had dealt with a similar incident where the baby had been badly affected. In the event of a serious incident involving a midwife, an SOM will undertake a supervisory enquiry on behalf of the Local Supervising Authority (LSA). On this occasion, there was no LSA enquiry, but the Labour Ward Coordinator met with Jen and Sue to talk through the incident. Sue had to console Jen, as it was a very difficult meeting. She felt quite wretched and devastated by her mistake, which could have had such far-reaching consequences.

Sue had to decide how best to help Jen. She knew that, to restore Jen's confidence, she would need some supported practice and a learning contract. Supported practice is a time-limited programme of working with the support of a supervisor but not under direct supervision. The midwife concerned meets regularly with the supervisor during the programme to discuss the women cared for and the care given. The midwife will also discuss the progress being made with his or her learning contract. In this particular case, the learning contract involved a record-keeping programme and CTG update, with a mentor for Jen to assist her with this. Sue asked Jen who she thought was the best person to be her mentor; it needed to be a midwife she respected who had good knowledge of record-keeping requirements and CTG. Jen chose the practice development midwife, who was delighted to help. The time limit for achieving all the aims of the learning contract was four weeks and, with Sue's support, Jen achieved all the aims and was able confidently to continue working on the labour ward.

Confidentiality was maintained throughout this process, with only Sue and the mentor being aware that Jen was working through a programme of supported practice. The regular meetings gave Jen a chance to discuss with Sue how she had come to terms with her error and how she felt she had learned, in fact benefited, from this. She was able to demonstrate a new confidence from her improved knowledge. The practice development midwife had completed CTG assessment with Jen and they were both pleased with the results. Jen's record keeping improved, as did her understanding of the need for accurate, contemporaneous records.

Sue didn't just leave Jen to it at the end of the learning contract, but she made regular informal contact to ensure that Jen was happy and confident in her work and knew that she was there if needed.

I hope that this vignette has demonstrated the positive response that supervision provides in the twenty-first century and how the SOM is there for the midwife through thick and thin. There are also plenty of examples of supervisors responding positively to midwives when they have done well, such as through new academic achievement or promotion. The supervisor is there to enjoy those good moments as well as the more difficult times.

Having a good relationship with your SOM from the start is essential to build up the belief in supervision that is needed to make it work. Sue, in the vignette, had made contact with Jen as soon as she started work at the maternity unit, when she was told that Jen had been allocated to her as an SOM. Sue knew Jen when she was a student midwife and was delighted when Jen chose her as her supervisor. They were slowly building a good relationship and Sue's aim was that this would be based on mutual respect.

Having an element of choice in the allocation of midwife to supervisor is essential, and that can work both ways, with the midwife choosing the supervisor and the supervisor choosing the supervisees. Usually, the midwife is invited to select three supervisors whom he or she would be happy to have as named SOM and the supervisor also has the opportunity to say 'No' if the list is already full or if the supervisor would not feel confident with that particular midwife–supervisor relationship.

Investigating critical incidents is not easy, no matter what the outcome. An SOM is well aware that, despite the blame culture that we appear to live in, no one deliberately tries to harm women or babies; perhaps the infamous nurse Beverley Allitt was the exception (Appleyard 1994). Similarly, no midwife is a fool; how could a fool qualify as a midwife? This means the supervisor's starting point in any enquiry must be 'what are the extenuating circumstances?'

Following a serious critical incident, there will inevitably be a management enquiry commissioned by the Trust through their risk management policy, but the supervisor acts independently of the Trust and on behalf of the LSA. It is not appropriate for the named SOM to undertake this enquiry as the supervisor needs to be available to support the midwife and listen to her or his account of events. Another SOM will be asked to undertake the supervisory enquiry on behalf of the LSA. The best approach is for the supervisor to get everyone together, meeting with all the midwives involved. It is very important to get the whole story from everyone at the same time, so that each midwife knows what happened when they were not in the birthing room. It helps everyone to get the true picture and to understand how the event developed.

Maintaining confidentiality is not easy when it is determined that supervised, rather than supported, practice is needed. When supervised practice is advocated, the midwife concerned must work all the time in a supernumerary capacity under the direct supervision of an SOM for a prescribed amount of time. This might seem harsh, but after a very serious incident the midwife's confidence can be badly knocked and he or she will feel more confident working with a supervisor. Similarly, the supervisor needs to know that the midwife can practise safely. As with supported practice, a robust learning programme runs in parallel, often with a midwifery lecturer providing academic support.

An old-fashioned response to a labour ward incident in many hospitals might have been to remove the midwife from the labour ward to work in the postnatal ward. But, just as getting back on your bike after falling off is the best approach, it is best to continue working in the same area. You cannot learn about best care in labour on a postnatal ward.

The vignette describes a hospital incident, but it could just as easily have been a home birth situation. Midwives value their role as autonomous practitioners and being able to work independently of medical staff in the home birth situation emphasises this more than anything else. It can be quite daunting for a midwife who is used to having plenty of people around in the hospital, especially the first home birth. There is an SOM available 24/7 in every area, so a midwife attending a home birth can contact the supervisor at any time for advice and a second opinion. Just having someone to bounce ideas off, especially when you are tired and/or stressed, can make a huge difference, and this kind of support is much appreciated by the midwife attending a home birth. Independent midwives who work mostly in the home environment also appreciate having an SOM at the other end of the telephone.

I deliberately chose a newly qualified midwife to use as an example in the vignette. The sudden change from student to qualified midwife has been mentioned elsewhere in this book but deserves further mention in a chapter on supervision. Although we welcome the autonomy of the midwife's role, it is the most challenging aspect of midwifery for the newly registered. Having been in a position of direct supervision and mentorship, the newly qualified midwife is expected to be capable of autonomous decision making overnight. Many have described this experience as being 'thrown into the lions' den'. Unfortunately, reduced staffing levels in many maternity units have led to newly qualified midwives being counted as pairs of hands on an understaffed shift, prohibiting well-managed preceptorship. Not many midwives can recount working alongside their preceptor on every shift in their first few weeks in post. The principle of preceptorship is to provide support and guidance for new registrants and enable them to make the transition from student to accountable practitioner (NMC 2006b). The newly qualified midwife should thus have protected learning time and access to, and regular meetings with, the preceptor for at least four months. The preceptor provides positive feedback of good performance and honest and objective feedback where performance could be improved, at the same time as facilitating new knowledge and skills. This is a tall order for any midwife working in a busy unit and on different shifts from the new registrant. With careful planning, however, it can work well and part of the SOM's first meeting with the newly qualified midwife will be to check that a preceptor has been allocated and that the relationship is working.

All this might seem an idyllic presentation of supervision, but this is how supervision can and does work. There will always be exceptions to the rule, especially where different personalities are involved. Each individual SOM will have different characteristics, but the guidance for supervisors is clear and easily available through many of the NMC publications, particularly the *Midwives Rules and Standards* (NMC 2004) and *Standards for the Preparation and Practice of Supervisors of Midwives* (NMC 2006a). There is also a lot of helpful material for midwives on how to make the most of supervision in *Modern Supervision in Action: A practical guide for midwives* (LSAMO/ NMC 2008).

Supervision has a very long history, being first introduced in 1902. More than 100 years later it continues to work effectively, with very few midwives being referred to the NMC (NMC 2004). It must, however, be used appropriately to be effective and it relies on a good relationship between the midwife and the SOM. It goes without saying that the supervision offered in 1902 was a far cry from that practised in 2009. The original style was very inspectoral and with good reason. We all remember Charles Dickens' apocryphal character, Sairey Gamp, in *Martin Chuzzlewit*, first published in 1844 (Dickens 1994). One cannot be sure that Dickens based her on a real-life midwife, but 60 years later there were still some very unsavoury midwives around and their inspection and regulation improved standards of care for women and babies.

For over 100 years, SOMs have been charged with protecting the public. Within recent years, however, the emphasis of the role has changed and supporting midwives is much more to the fore. It stands to reason, though, that if a midwife is supported she is less likely to perform sub-optimally, is more likely to seek advice when she is unsure about a situation and is more likely to ask for help when needed.

The SOM is also there for the mothers, but it has always proved difficult to get this message across to women whose first contact is with the midwife. They are unlikely to have contact, or need contact, with an SOM if all goes well in their programme of care. Sadly, it is usually only when something goes wrong, or when her needs are not being met, that a woman learns about the role of the supervisor. To address this, the NMC has recently published a leaflet called *Support for Parents: How supervision and supervisors of midwives can help you* (NMC 2008).

Whether a midwife is newly qualified or has been practising for many years, he or she will still value the annual review with the SOM. This is a protected, personal time for the midwife for a reflective review of his or her midwifery practice during the previous year. Aspirations for the coming year can be discussed and the supervisor's support can be sought in providing learning opportunities to achieve those aspirations. Any concerns about practice can be discussed in this confidential arena, secure in the knowledge that the supervisor is in a position to offer support and guidance and take action where needed.

It is not intended to give the impression that midwives should be totally dependent on their SOM. Far from it, overdependence would be a trial to the supervisor and would not assist the midwife in personal development. Ideally, the supervisory relationship should be one of empowerment and this can only be achieved if there is a respect for supervision and the supervisor.

The SOM is also a practising midwife and, although many midwifery managers are SOMs, the majority are clinical midwives. This means that the supervisors have their own dilemmas in clinical practice and need the help and support of their own supervisors. Supervision is part of the wonderful chain of 'caring for the carers' within midwifery. The mother cares for her baby, the midwife cares for the mother, the SOM cares for the midwife and the supervisor's SOM cares for him or her.

The LSA Midwifery Officer (LSAMO) is responsible for the supervision of midwives within a particular area. There are 16 LSAMOs in the UK covering large areas. They visit each Trust annually to monitor the supervision and standards of midwifery and supervisory practice. Despite covering such huge areas with thousands of midwives, they can still be approached by individual midwives or parents if they feel that supervision is not being carried out appropriately in their area or if there are any concerns about midwifery practice that the caller believes are not being addressed. The LSAMO will then investigate accordingly.

Supervision, as with any aspect of any profession, may have had its criticisms. This could, perhaps, be due to misunderstanding the role. The recent LSAMO/NMC publication (2008) aims to resolve those misunderstandings. One of those misunderstandings is regarding the LSAMO having the power to suspend a midwife from practice. This is not something that happens frequently and is also confused with suspension from duty. The former can only be done by an LSAMO and refers to preventing a midwife from practising anywhere, while the latter refers to a Trust preventing a midwife from working in the Trust pending a disciplinary hearing. These powers are needed in order to protect the public, but are rarely used.

Another misunderstanding is that supervisors are there to inspect and criticise. It is interesting that, early in the last century, the Central Midwives Board advised that the SOM should be a 'friend and counsellor' rather than a 'relentless critic' (MoH 1937).

Supervisors are certainly expected to monitor midwifery practice, but criticism should be constructive and helpful and the response to any incident should be proactive rather than reactive and punitive. That proactive response must also be appropriate, hence the two levels of response to serious incidents: supported practice or supervised practice. The majority of supervision is undertaken without either action and I hope I have described how it can have a very positive effect on midwifery practice and midwives.

Commentary

On the basis of her wealth of experience as a supervisor, Jean provides a fundamentally real picture of what midwifery supervision is all about. As she mentions, there are many different meanings of the word 'supervision'. It may include the clinical supervision that our nursing cousins have sought to implement as a form of quality control. In the areas of counselling and mental health nursing, though, supervision assumes more of a psychodynamic function.

So how does midwifery supervision relate to these occupational groups, which, though different, may not be a million miles away from midwifery in its woman-centred orientation?

The answer comes out of Jean's chapter in two ways. The first is in the form of the potential for supervision to enhance the midwife's practice and, thus, the childbearing experience of the woman for whom she or he cares. The second is found in the midwife's perception of being supported, which makes the midwife better able to provide truly supportive care for the woman by being able to engage healthily with her at the depth the woman requires. In this way, the chain of caring for carers to which Jean refers manifests itself.

Although it is clear that the SOM is perfectly positioned to undertake these roles in a formalised way, the question arises whether any informal mechanisms exist to provide similar functions. The answer is clearly 'Yes', in that midwives interact with and support each other in their casual and interpersonal encounters. These contacts may comprise little more than a fleeting encounter in the corridor or in the street. A few casual words may be sufficient to express an interest in well-being that constitutes support. Similarly, a chance meeting in the coffee-room may permit an opportunity to mull over a challenging situation or some other 'unfinished business'. More explicitly, there is the spontaneous 'Let's all go to the pub' reaction after a particularly unfortunate event or difficult shift. In such situations, a slightly strange form of humour may manifest itself. To outsiders, such humour may appear objectionable to the point of being macabre or possibly dangerous, but, to the group who are involved, it serves to bind together colleagues facing common difficulties (Sullivan 2000).

References

Appleyard, W.J. (1994) 'Murder in the NHS', *British Medical Journal* 308, 29 January: 287–8.

Dickens, C. (1994) *Martin Chuzzlewit*, Ware: Wordsworth Editions.

LSA Midwifery Officers National (UK) Forum/Nursing and Midwifery Council (LSAMO/NMC) (2008) *Modern Supervision in Action: A practical guide for midwives*, London: NMC.

Ministry of Health (MoH) (1937) *Supervision of Midwives*, Circular 1620, London: MoH.

Nursing and Midwifery Council (NMC) (2004) *Midwives Rules and Standards*, London: NMC.

Nursing and Midwifery Council (NMC) (2006a) *Standards for the Preparation and Practice of Supervisors of Midwives*, London: NMC.

Nursing and Midwifery Council (NMC) (2006b) *Preceptorship Guidelines*, London: NMC.

Nursing and Midwifery Council (NMC) (2008) *Support for Parents: How supervision and supervisors of midwives can help you*, London: NMC.

Sullivan, E. (2000) 'Gallows humour in social work practice: an issue for supervision and reflexivity', *Practice* 12(2): 45–54.

Chapter 8

The academic midwife

Rosemary Mander

Working in the postnatal ward, I was allocated to take over the care of Fiona, who had given birth to Morag two days earlier. Alison, the midwife from the morning shift, was introducing me to Fiona and telling me about the progress she and Morag were making. I soon realised I'd seen Fiona before, but could not recall where.

Alison introduced me by my first name, saying that I'd be caring for Fiona and Morag during the evening. To our surprise, Fiona demanded to know what I was doing there and whether I'd be doing research on her or using her for teaching.

I quickly realised that I'd seen Fiona at various educational meetings, because she was a lecturer at another local university. Alison tried to explain that I regularly 'volunteered' to work on the ward, sharing all aspects of the work with the other midwives and that, if any of 'my' university's students were on the ward, I would work with them, but that did not apply that day.

Fiona accepted Alison's explanation and later we discussed this pattern of work, which was clearly quite new to Fiona. While we agreed that there could be benefits for all involved, this encounter made me think carefully about what it is that the academic midwife does.

Introduction

Being a midwife working in an academic setting may sound idyllic. In many ways this is the perfect job. As a midwife, I find the freedom to organise my own work and pursue my own occupational interests incredible. In this section, though, I reflect on how this occupational freedom may be used and whether there are any other ways in which it may be interpreted.

Having been employed in the health service for approximately 15 years of my 40-odd-year working life, and having worked in it for a great majority of my working life, I consider myself to be in a position to compare work in the two settings. These comparisons are likely to recur throughout this section.

How did I get to where I am?

The background that I have outlined already probably raises the question of how and why this move into academia happened. The immediate answer is 'Much to my own surprise!' This disbelief is largely due to my having been written off at an early stage as 'not university material', which I accepted as an objective and authoritative assessment of my intellectual ability.

A more considered answer, though, reflects a searching for a way to influence the care that is provided for the childbearing woman and her baby. As was quite usual at that time, having completed nurse training I found myself effectively railroaded into midwifery. It was as a result of inertia, more than any active decision on my part, that I found myself in midwifery practice. After practising in a number of different settings, I realised that I was only able to influence the care of the women within my own rather limited sphere of practice. I recognised that I had little opportunity to change ideas about midwifery care in more general terms.

On this basis, I concluded that educating the next generation of midwives would be the way to make a difference to the provision of midwifery care. So I became a midwifery teacher, responsible for a small school educating midwives for a group of three maternity units in the north-east of England. It did not take me long to grasp that the student midwives' education was but one of a wide range of factors that may influence the care that midwives offer.

It became clear to me that what was necessary was to find out more about that care and the system within which the childbearing woman receives teaching, support and nurturing from the midwife. To do this, research would be needed and this required me to move into the higher education (HE) sector.

In this setting, I was comfortable with my teaching role, and I soon started to come to terms with the challenges of research. The need for, and opportunities presented by, writing and publication probably should not have come as such a surprise. These latter aspects of my work have become my major focus. Perhaps fortuitously, in the institution in which I am employed, the route to promotion has traditionally been largely through research and publication.

With the benefit of hindsight, it may be that I was naive to assume that there might be one single solution to the challenge of providing appropriate and effective care to the childbearing woman. I now believe that the challenge is complex to the point of being a conundrum. There have been suggestions that systemic problems inherent in maternity units might be addressed by augmenting the community midwifery and home birth services. This change has long been introduced in countries such as New Zealand, but the increasing rates of medical intervention there do not appear to have been remedied (NZHIS 2003). In the UK, the move towards community-based midwifery is happening at an almost imperceptibly slow rate, despite midwife-led care having been shown to be effective in a number of centres (Walsh 2006). The complexity of the challenge is recognised in the writing of one academic midwife who considers that a combination of roles in the form of the consultant midwife will provide the answer (Kirkman 2007).

What does the academic midwife actually do?

One problem with the word 'academic' is that its link with 'freedom' may be unrealistically firm in the minds of those who have never experienced being an academic. For this reason, my move into HE brought with it an undisguised awareness of my own autonomy. Academic freedom has been defined in terms of no interference by academic or external authorities in the scholar's teaching, researching, publishing, speaking or writing (Kayrooz and Preston 2002). Such freedom incorporates an inherent momentum, which serves to motivate or to drive the individual. This drive operates in spite of the widely held assumption that academic life is one long, lazy, sun-drenched sabbatical.

As well as enjoying this relative freedom, academics are also required to complete their contractual obligations to their employing institution. Although contracts of employment vary between higher education institutions (HEIs), my contract requires that I should teach and research, together with completing the associated administrative work. As shown in the vignette, the proportions of each of these activities will vary with institutions, individuals and workload. Perhaps because the administrative tasks are something we would all rather forget about, I will focus on the research and teaching aspects of my role. Academics are encouraged to endeavour to ensure that these two aspects are interdependent; for me the result is that my teaching emerges largely out of my (as well as others') research. Reciprocally, questions that arise out of my teaching serve to feed into and stimulate my programme of research.

This interdependence between teaching and research, though, has a tendency to neglect the crucial role that clinical practice plays in the life of the academic midwife. My vignette shows how my practice has been facilitated by an honorary contract with a local maternity unit. This contract has permitted me to work as a midwife 'without status', as my contract states, in the labour ward and in ante- and postnatal settings (Mander 1992). Both childbearing women and clinical colleagues have found it difficult to understand this clinical input. But I don't believe that it is possible to overstate the significance of clinical practice to the academic midwife. This significance may be appropriately summed up in terms of the 'three Rs'.

Research

Clinical practice permits the academic midwife to stay involved with 'grass roots' clinical activity and ideas. In this way, practice that is (or is not) changing may suggest lines of study. An example that, admittedly, predates my move into academia was my observation, when I was a midwife tutor, of the attrition among newly qualified midwives. This observation led to my doctoral research (Mander 1993a). Similarly, and more recently, I observed the 'rugger pass approach' to the care of a mother relinquishing her baby for adoption. This observation led to my research examining the care of this woman and comparisons between her care and that of the bereaved mother (Mander 2006).

Writing

In the same way that research ideas may be stimulated by clinical practice, ideas for publications also arise. This happens with thoughts that need to be aired or discussed, but that may be at too early a stage to justify research. Thus, some journal editors may welcome opinion pieces. The author, effectively, has the opportunity to 'run an idea up the flagpole – to find out whether anybody salutes it'. An example is a paper examining the issues relating to breastfeeding promotion (Mander 2008).

Reality

It has been known for universities to be criticised for being like 'ivory towers'. This criticism of elitism may possibly occasionally be justified. Such criticisms have no place in the context of the practice disciplines, such as midwifery. Clinical practice permits me, as an academic, to keep my feet well and truly on the ground. This is crucial for the other components of the academic role, such as research, administration and, particularly, teaching.

Summarising what the academic midwife actually does

These aforementioned 'three Rs' serve to combine together into an overarching function of the academic midwife. This function may be summarised quite simply as 'questioning'. As I have said already, these questions may take the form of research projects and publications in the form of books or articles in journals.

Might the questioning take other forms, though? Obviously the answer is going to be 'Yes'. But this answer may not be so obvious when it is remembered that academics are widely regarded as knowledgeable in quite specific ways. Some may assume that an academic, by virtue of that title, will automatically be able to provide an answer to any query – no matter how obscure. In the middle of a busy labour ward I have been asked 'Rosemary, tell me the names of all of the learning styles.' Equally inappropriately, I have been asked 'What exactly is Ogilvie's syndrome, Rosemary?'

The academic midwife's questioning may well arise out of her clinical practice, as in my example (above) of the care of a mother relinquishing her baby for adoption. Other questions may be less acceptable or more controversial to the point of being heretical. An example might be my questioning of the increasing use of epidural analgesia in labour (Mander 1993b, 1994) or the benefits of men being involved in childbirth (Mander 2004). Such questions matter because they encourage the thinking of uncomfortable, even unthinkable, thoughts.

These kinds of questions, though, tend not to make the academic midwife's life easy. In a culture that values providing answers, asking difficult questions might not be universally welcomed. Similarly, in a health care system that is medically dominated there may be a certain in-built conservatism. In such situations it may be considered important for all to be 'singing from the same hymn sheet'. Thus, because the NHS is a setting in which conformity is highly prized, unanswerable questions that threaten to disrupt the status quo may be given a distinctly cool reception. This midwife's movement between two settings with very different attitudes to questioning does not make for an easy life.

Such reactions lead to thoughts of what this means to the individual academic midwife.

What does it mean to be an academic midwife?

While there are clearly benefits to working in an academic setting, it may be emerging, though, that there could be a downside to this idyllic picture. Some of these drawbacks relate to the fundamental nature of midwifery as a practice discipline. The contrast between the 'hands-on' nature of midwifery and the more abstract approach of academia may occasionally be discomforting. This is because the academic midwife needs to, effectively, maintain 'a foot in both camps', if she or he is to retain any degree of credibility with those who work and practise alongside. This credibility matters because midwives cannot allow themselves or their input to be written off by either their academic or their midwifery practitioner colleagues. This would constitute a disaster in personal as well as occupational terms. Thus, the academic midwife may have to work twice as hard as colleagues whose disciplines may be even more firmly embedded in academia.

It is understandable that this slightly schizoid existence may occasionally be less than comfortable. Any discomfort may be aggravated, though, by a fundamental lack of understanding among colleagues in both settings. In academia, midwifery could easily be dismissed as simply practical, even manual, tasks. This ease of dismissal may be aggravated by the difficulty of explaining what midwives *actually* do to ensure that childbirth and childbearing remain within the parameters of normality. Because midwives may not be able to articulate the complexity of what it means to be 'with woman', others may cast aspersions, suggesting that clinical practice is little more than 'bedpans, bags and tubes'. Thus, academic colleagues may be dismissive or, even worse, patronising about the clinical component of midwifery.

While academics may have a hard time understanding what midwifery is about, the same may also be true of clinical colleagues' perceptions of academic life. This may be because some influential middle-grade midwives have had a limited experience of university education. For this reason, the 'ivory tower' image may still prevail. Such images may constitute the uncomfortable basis of misunderstandings. It is possible that the move of midwifery education into HEIs may have remedied these misperceptions. I do sometimes get the impression, though, that students regard the academic role as solely one of formal teaching. So it may be that news of this remedy has been somewhat exaggerated. Another aspect of such misunderstandings is explored in the Conclusion to this book (page 217).

A further issue the academic midwife faces, and that may not be unrelated to the issues mentioned already, relates to the title itself. By this I mean that 'academic' has been known to be used as, if not a term of abuse, at least a disparaging one. On these occasions, 'academic' may be preceded by 'simply', 'purely' or 'only' or may be followed by 'pedantry', 'nicety' or 'argument'. The reasons for 'academic' being used in this way may be associated with the relatively low status of social scientists and health scholars compared with certain other occupational groups. With regard to its more general use, it may reflect a rather obtuse, even inverted, form of snobbery.

The meaning of being an academic midwife clearly has its negative aspects. These should in no way outweigh the good news. As well as the perceptions mentioned already of making a difference in a broad-brush as well as long-term approach, there is also the occasional frisson of pure delight. Such blissful moments occur when it becomes plain, occasionally in rather unlikely settings, that the work of the academic midwife is being read and may even yet be acted on. Such ego-boosting experiences include the occasional disbelieving question from a clinician or student along the lines of 'Are you *the* Rosemary Mander?'

Similarly, students' views may change. This includes the student who is healthily critical of, to the point of vehemently opposing, the ideas presented as part of the curriculum. This may include my praise of my clinical midwifery colleagues for their ability to be 'with women'. Such opposition, even ridicule, is obliterated when years later that former student admits:

- 'I didn't believe you then.'
- 'I was convinced that you were wrong.'
- 'I realise now that you were right all along.'

Conclusion

In this reflection on my role as an academic midwife, an aspect that has emerged quite prominently is the differences and disharmonies between the HE environment and the clinical environment. With further reflection, it may be helpful to contemplate, and perhaps to qualify, the development of these differences.

As those working in it know only too well, the HE sector has undergone a series of immeasurable changes since the middle of the twentieth century. There is no reason to believe that, at the beginning of the twenty-first century, these changes are complete. Similarly, since its inception in 1946 (MoH 1946) the changes in the NHS have been persistent, painful and colossal.

The transformations in these two massive sectors may have had a certain amount in common. One aspect that is certainly common to both organisations is the move towards commercialisation. In the HE sector the generation of income has come to depend on teaching programmes and on individuals and groups of researchers. In the health care system, income generation has impinged even more directly on the consumers of the services.

On the basis of these developments, I would like to suggest that the role of the academic midwife is likely, as these two organisations become more closely comparable, to become less challenging. Or it may be that the challenges will only assume different forms.

Commentary

As a fellow midwife academic, I was immediately struck by the words 'Being a midwife working in an academic setting may sound idyllic' in this chapter. My first thought was 'how could anyone ever think that?' However, standing back and taking time to reflect on these words, together with Rosemary's supporting rationale for the kind of work we do, I realise that to some midwives it may indeed seem idyllic.

Officially we do not work unsociable hours, we can carry out research in our areas of interest and we can shape the next genera- tions of midwives to come. These tasks, however, carry a considerable deal of responsibility and one of the strongest messages we need to give out is that of encouraging healthy debate and critique. Rosemary speaks of the notion of universities as ivory towers and, indeed, a question still often asked is 'why do midwives need to be trained in universities?'

My response, and indeed that of Rosemary, is that it is through universities that the midwives of the future will engage in critique and drive the profession forward, instead of being subservient to medicine and in some cases being replaced by nurses. A healthy professional foundation at bachelor's level is also essential, so that midwives are orientated to the notion of academia and a proportion will go on to become the next generation of academics.

References

Kayrooz, C. and Preston, P. (2002) 'Academic freedom: impressions of Australian social scientists', *Minerva* 40: 341–58.

Kirkman, S. (2007) 'Reflections on midwifery by the recently retired', *The Practising Midwife* 10(11): 15–16.

Mander, R. (1992) 'The value of clinical experience to a non-clinician: combining midwifery practice with teaching', *Midwifery* 8(4): 184–90.

Mander, R. (1993a) 'Midwifery training and the years after qualification', in Robinson, S. and Thomson, A. (eds) *Midwives, Research and Childbirth*, London: Routledge.

Mander, R. (1993b) 'Epidural analgesia 1: recent history', *British Journal of Midwifery* 1(6): 259–64.

Mander, R. (1994) 'Epidural analgesia: 2: research basis', *British Journal of Midwifery* 2(1): 12–16.

Mander, R. (2004) *Men and Maternity*, London: Routledge.

Mander, R. (2006) *Loss and Bereavement in Childbearing*, 2nd edition, London: Routledge.

Mander, R. (2008) 'Baby friendly – mother friendly? Policy issues in breastfeeding promotion', *MIDIRS* 18(1): 104–6 and 108.

Ministry of Health (MoH) (1946) *National Health Service Bill: Summary of the proposed new service*, Ministry of Health Cmd 6761, London: HMSO.

New Zealand Health Information Service (NZHIS) (2003) *Report on Maternity 2000 and 2001*, Wellington: New Zealand Ministry of Health.

Walsh, D. (2006) *Improving Maternity Services: Small is beautiful: lessons for maternity services from a birth centre*, Oxford: Radcliffe Publishing.

Chapter 9

The midwife as a researcher

Ans Luyben

Introduction

Once you have become a midwife, being a researcher is not the first thing that comes to your mind. Midwifery is an exciting profession. It is fascinating how a new life begins, and the individuality of a woman's experience is challenging. Newly qualified midwives, therefore, will primarily choose to work with pregnant women, their children and families in everyday practice. Practising midwifery not only involves scientific knowledge, but also art and caring sensitivity, in which midwives use their own personality in order to achieve positive effects in caring for mothers and their families. While these magic elements are essential to care, they have been hard to capture and evaluate in studies (Enkin and Chalmers 1982). In everyday practice, however, midwives are often confronted with standardising, medical research. Many midwives have experienced this kind of research, in contrast to the individual approach needed for their work. Being a researcher, therefore, seems like following a different profession. Midwifery research addresses midwives' ways of working and aims to improve midwifery practice. If this happens, research can be as fascinating as midwifery. Well-known midwife researchers started their first research with a question that arose from practice, and thus contributed to the reduction of unnecessary interventions during childbirth.

My research career started when I questioned aspects of practice during my training and experienced the difference that research can make. Our research project on parameters for diagnosing intrauterine growth retardation (slow growth in babies) led to a reduction in the numbers of hormone measurements in the hospital in which I worked. Motivated by this outcome, my next question again arose in practice and resulted in a reduction in adverse outcomes of breech birth (Roumen and Luyben 1991). From these experiences I learnt about the importance of research evidence for practice, as well as its compatibility with the art of midwifery.

Meanwhile, midwifery research has developed. One of its greatest current strengths is the rich diversity of methods (Cluett and Bluff 2003). This diversity in particular allows midwives currently not only to address the medical, but also several other aspects of midwifery practice. The objectives of this research, as well as a short history of midwifery researchers, are described in the next sections. Thereafter, a picture of the role of a midwife as a researcher is presented, based on the literature, personal information from midwife researchers in the UK and the United States of America (USA) and my own experience, as well as the current experiences of three midwives doing research in three European countries: Mechthild (Germany), Greta (the Netherlands) and Martina (Switzerland).

Why midwifery research is needed

Throughout history, midwifery knowledge had most often been orally transferred from midwife to midwife and little was documented. This way, knowledge was discovered and developed, but also lost. Only a few midwives left their knowledge in a written form, such as Catharina Schrader, who documented her midwifery experiences in the Netherlands during the eighteenth century as case studies (van Lieburg 1984). Until the second half of the twentieth century, however, midwifery knowledge was mainly based on authority, tradition, intuition, experience and research by other disciplines.

A call for midwifery research was raised during the 1970s and 1980s, particularly in the USA and the UK. Professional questioning of the effectiveness of maternity care, as well as the involvement of consumers, indicated the need for childbirth reforms. This development coincided with the establishment of the profession of nurse-midwives in the USA and the search for recognition of their care. Meanwhile, medical professionals in the UK aimed to reduce maternal and perinatal mortality and morbidity and increase the effectiveness of interventions in maternity care through systematic evaluation, which also involved midwifery (Chalmers *et al.* 1989). As a result, the need for basing professional practice on research was emphasised.

Midwifery research aims, therefore, to create a body of midwifery knowledge, which underpins and improves midwifery practice, and thus maternity care, which involves:

- improving the effectiveness and quality of maternity care, which includes the provision of woman-centred care;
- expanding knowledge of the multiple aspects of a woman's childbearing process (for example, physiological, psychological, sociological), as well as the influence of maternity care on this process;
- increasing the number of options for maternity care available to women;
- increasing evidence-based practice and developing standards of maternity care;
- developing a sound basis, as well as vision, for midwifery practice.

A short history of midwives as researchers

Midwifery research and the professional role of a researcher only go back about three decades. Before this time, new knowledge was merely generated by researchers in other disciplines, in particular obstetrics and nursing. Reva Rubin, for example, developed a nursing theory of becoming a mother during the 1970s. In a similar way, the active management of labour is based on research from medical practitioners. Several researchers, such as the team of the World Health Organisation (WHO), stressed, however, the need for mid-wives to conduct research in their own field. Following a study of maternity services in Europe during the 1970s, they stated:

midwives have to study the work of midwives, together with competent scientists, so that they gradually create a body of explicit midwifery knowledge and raise a group of midwifery researchers. Part of this research has to be qualitative [focusing on the everyday experience of people and using methods such as interviews and observations] and will hopefully question the contribution of lay and traditionally trained midwives to maternity care.

(WHO 1987: 93)

Posts for midwifery researchers were first established in English-speaking countries, although the integration of research as a professional role and topics of research varied in these countries. In the USA, research focused on proving the effectiveness of midwifery care, including home birth, birth centres and care for vulnerable groups (Farley 2005). Some midwives documented their practical experience, such as Ina May Gaskin, who systematically evaluated 82 cases of using the All-Fours Manoeuvre for reducing problems with birthing the shoulders of the baby during labour (Bruner et al. 1998). In the UK, recognition of midwives as researchers particularly increased as some midwives used research to challenge issues of their everyday practice. A well-known pioneer was Jennifer Sleep, who studied the liberal performance of episiotomies (incisions into the soft tissues of the birth outlet) in a randomised controlled trial during the 1980s, while being supported by researchers from the Perinatal Epidemiology Unit in Oxford. The results showed that the number of episiotomies during labour could be reduced. Other examples of topics addressed by midwife researchers during the 1980s were the provision of information by midwives during labour (Kirkham 1989) and pushing techniques in the second stage of labour (Thomson 1993).

In other European countries, this development happened later and was supported by research workshops held by midwives from the UK. In some countries, midwives succeeded in doing research as part of a postgraduate study. In Sweden, Gunny Röckner (Röckner et al. 1989) carried out a doctoral study on the frequency of episiotomies and spontaneous tears close to her retirement, although she had wanted to do research for most of her professional life. Some undertook research as members of an interdisciplinary teams. In the Netherlands, Rita Iedema-Kuiper (1996) did a doctoral study, in cooperation with researchers from other disciplines, on the effectiveness of home care for women with a high-risk pregnancy. Other midwives documented their experiences or carried out small research projects in midwifery practice. In Austria, Gaby Sprung (1998) studied the use of medicine during labour, and found that a trusting relationship between midwife and woman reduced its frequency. Another important topic implemented and studied in several countries with midwives as researchers was the model of a midwife-led unit.

Current places of work of midwife researchers

The availability of the post of midwife researcher varies per country. Some countries, such as the UK or the Netherlands, have professional or national guidelines describing the need for midwives to conduct research and mentioning this role, whereas in other countries this role is established as part of a research appointment for a master's degree or doctoral study, or has to be created. After completing her doctorate, Mechthild in Germany found a combined post of working as a midwife and being a research fellow under the Head of the Department of Obstetrics and Gynaecology of a German hospital. She created her new post herself and developed it into being a midwife researcher in practice, although this is still unique in Germany.

Midwives are working as researchers in different practical settings, most often, however, in large tertiary hospitals. Some midwives work as research midwives, while carrying out research projects as their main occupation. These posts vary slightly depending on the kind of clinical projects involved, who is leading the project, the funding source, and whether the midwife is also working in practice or education. Greta in the Netherlands thus works three days a week on a doctoral project as a Research Midwife at a university hospital and one day as a midwife in clinical practice. Other midwives are doing research as an integral part of their posts, which include Practice Development Midwife, Consultant Midwife or Midwifery Expert, such as Martina in a Swiss university hospital. Her work includes improving evidence-based practice, developing standards of midwifery care, organising courses for midwives in the hospital and carrying out research projects in cooperation with the Department of Clinical Research.

Midwives also work as researchers in other health care organisations and institutions in midwifery-specific domains, as well as being members of interdisciplinary teams. Examples of such organisations and institutions are NHS Trusts (UK), governmental or regional Health Departments, various Institutes for Health Technology Assessment, and the Netherlands Institute for Health Services Research (NIVEL).

Training

Postgraduate training should provide midwife researchers with the methodological and methodical competencies they need for carrying out research projects, which involves theory as well as practical experience. Before the establishment of research as a professional role for midwives in the UK, they had to identify the relevant courses themselves and most training was self-funded and had to be attended in personal time. Currently, this training is likely to be considered integral to the role and to be funded. A similar trend can be noticed in other European countries.

Some agreement exists that the minimum requirement for training to prepare midwives for the role of midwife researcher consists of study at master's level (M.Sc. or M.Phil.), which includes research and a research dissertation. Both Greta and Mechthild completed a master's degree on a part-time basis and funded it themselves. Greta's doctoral study is an integral part of her current post. Whereas Martina had already started a part-time, self-funded Master's in Midwifery, time to finish this study is an integral part of the post. The availability of the required training, however, varies per country, as in many countries a midwifery-specific master's degree is not offered. Alternative training involves studying abroad (probably in the UK or USA), studying in another discipline (for example, public health or nursing) or attending several relevant postgraduate courses in research (for example, Certificate of Advanced Studies or Diploma of Advanced Studies).

Salary

As the post of the midwife researcher is not officially established in all countries, the salary varies. The main influencing factor is the national system of remuneration. Additional factors that play a role in regard to the salary in the three different countries discussed here involve the job description, working experience as a midwife and the level of study required for the post. Most salaries are a bit higher than those of midwives in practice, due to the higher requirements in regard to training. In some posts the salaries of researchers increase depending on the acquisition of external finances.

Everyday work

The structure of a day in the life of a midwife researcher depends on the job description. A midwife doing research as an integral part of a post (for example, Practice Development Midwife) will have a different structure of working day than a researcher who is working on a project full-time. This researcher might have his or her own project, but also work as a member of a larger team. Like Greta in the Netherlands, the researcher usually has their own project plan to follow in an autonomous, and sometimes also solitary way. However, participation in a few other projects is also likely, while working together with obstetricians, neonatologists, epidemiologists and midwives.

A normal day might be working from nine to five, but, depending on the project plan and the stage of the project, it might also involve working late or even being on call. Such a day, for example while working on a clinical trial in the postnatal ward, might involve discussing the research with women, seeing whether there are any new research participants, collecting clinical samples and data, documenting these data, reading related research papers and discussing the study with colleagues or students. Whereas a clinical trial might involve collecting clinical samples and data in the hospital, a qualitative study could involve interviewing women at home. A lot of time in research is also involved in analysing data, documenting the study and writing up the results. For some midwife researchers their working day might also involve acquisition of new projects with external funding, as well as professional development related to the project and/or their post.

Depending on the position of the midwife researcher in the hospital, sometimes other clinical staff activities (meetings, audits, presentations) are integrated in the working day. As a Midwifery Expert, Martina in Switzerland has a variety of clinical roles integrated in her job. Therefore, her everyday activities involve counselling colleagues, evaluating case studies of midwifery care, developing, implementing and evaluating practice programmes and standards and, of course, research.

Projects

The post of a midwife researcher in practice is often related to an institution's objectives to initiate research projects in midwifery and obstetrics/gynaecology, or to an existing project (or part of a project) that needs to be carried out by a midwife researcher. Mechthild, for example, pursued her doctoral project on influential factors on the birth process, such as the rupture of membranes or pain relief, in her new job, and she managed to involve a few other regional hospitals. Greta's study investigates if the current model of auditing cases of perinatal mortality and morbidity is an adequate representation of the quality of maternity care. Her project does not only involve data from the hospital she works in, but from the whole country. Both projects are financed by the researchers' hospitals, although Mechthild's post also involves the acquisition of external funding.

Many small projects are (and have been) carried out by midwives doing research as an integral part of their posts. The questions for these projects arise directly from midwifery practice and directly feed back into it. For these smaller projects, financing is often not a particular issue, as midwives are working on them as part of their job. Some projects initiated in practice might, however, expand, as does the research role of the midwife. A good example of such projects has been the implementation of the midwife-led unit. Turnbull *et al.* (1996) evaluated the outcomes of midwife-led care compared with traditional care during labour for low-risk women in a Scottish hospital. The study concluded that this model of care was clinically effective, and that women in the midwife-led unit had the same or lower rate of interventions and were more satisfied than women in traditional care. Following this study, several midwife-led units were implemented in other European countries (Austria, Switzerland and Germany) (Schuster 1998; Cignacco *et al.* 2004; Bauer and zu Sayn-Wittgenstein 2006). As this new model of care was a political issue in these countries, the implementation of the unit had to be accompanied by research, and this thus raised the need for midwife researchers.

The projects mentioned above are only a few examples of research carried out by midwives in practice. A complete overview of international midwifery research is hard to create, due to the fact that midwives are not always the lead researchers, and they also participate in the research projects of medical practitioners and collect samples (such as blood or amniotic liquid) or data during their work in the birthing room. Following the development and establishment of the professional role of the midwife in research, however, the Midwifery Research Database was initiated in the UK. The publication *MIRIAD* (Simms *et al.* 1994), based on the data collected in this database, provides an overview of midwifery research projects carried out in the UK during recent decades, and is a good example of the documentation of professional research by midwives.

Networking and cooperation

Networks are essential for doing midwifery research for a variety of reasons. Primarily, they are necessary for gaining direct support for doing one's own research, which involves having access to experts for counselling, as well as statistical and computer support. In some countries, this support network is available in the institutions where research takes place, whereas in other countries researchers have to create it themselves, which is often associated with extra costs. Without such a supporting network, however, it is almost impossible to carry out a research project.

A second reason for needing a network is the opportunity to discuss the study, knowledge exchange in regard to the research topic, and dissemination of the results of the study. Being located in university hospitals, Martina and Mechthild, as well as Greta, work together with midwifery, medical and research colleagues, and have the opportunity for the presentation of their study, and for discussion and exchange. Greta's network even goes beyond the hospital setting, and involves several national and international working groups on auditing maternity care, particularly perinatal statistics.

Conferences also provide a good platform for the dissemination of a study, and in particular for getting to know, and discuss with, other researchers who are addressing a similar topic. Another valuable international platform for presenting one's study, discussing it with midwifery colleagues and getting expert opinions is the Midwifery Research List (www.jiscmail.ac.uk). Some countries have created their own platform for midwifery research. For example, midwifery schools in the Netherlands have created a national web-based platform. Kennispoort Verloskunde (www.kennispoort-verloskunde.nl) not only provides an overview of midwifery research, but also of studies in maternity care carried out by researchers from other disciplines.

Careers

As the role of the midwife as a researcher is a rather new phenomenon, little is known about career possibilities. The careers of the earliest midwife researchers in the UK were related to the new professional orientation of midwifery. Some found a post within research units affiliated with universities or large health care institutions, such as the Perinatal Epidemiology Unit in Oxford. Others took up a post in a university as a lecturer, researcher or head of a midwifery school or department of health sciences. Best known are the midwife researchers who became professors, either through the need for professors in midwifery as a result of moving into HE, or through a step-wise academic career in research and education.

Other possible careers for midwife researchers involve management in a hospital, such as head of a department, or management or expert positions in health care institutions or organisations, for example the WHO. Because it is such a new role, new jobs might develop that cannot be imagined at this moment or, as one of the midwife researchers in this chapter wrote in regard to her career, 'the future will tell.'

Many thanks to Mechthild Gross, Martina Gisin, Helen Spiby and Greta Rijninks-van Driel for sharing their experiences.

Commentary

Becoming a midwife researcher is, as shown in this chapter, a career that involves a lot of study and patience. Although in their initial education many midwives are now required to have an understanding of the research process, it is not until the postgraduate programmes (usually at doctoral level) are undertaken that a midwife learns to become a researcher.

It is therefore not surprising that, as Ans points out, there are few midwives who consider themselves as researchers, although in Chapter 8 Rosemary has also highlighted research as an issue pertinent to the academic midwife. To be in the fortunate position of being a midwife researcher is a luxury of which many midwives only dream.

However, the research world is cut-throat at times and many researchers (both midwives and others) are required to earn their salaries from external funding. This involves many hours of filling in applications to various funding bodies, often with unsuccessful outcomes. To be a midwife researcher, therefore, requires considerable patience and an optimistic outlook.

Ans has also highlighted one of the main strengths of the job, as true interdisciplinary working as an equal partner, and this is vital when remembering that the main beneficiaries of our research must be the childbearing woman.

References

Bauer, N. and Sayn-Wittgenstein, F. zu (2006) 'Hebammenkreißsaal: Besonderheiten eines randomisiert, kontrollierten Studiendesigns', *Die Hebamme* 19(2): 107–19.

Bruner, J.P., Drummond, S., Meenan, A.I. and Gaskin, I.M. (1998) 'The all-fours manoeuvre for reducing shoulder dystocia during labour', *Journal of Reproductive Medicine* 43: 433–9.

Chalmers, I., Enkin, M. and Keirse, M.J.N.C. (1989) *Effective Care in Pregnancy and Childbirth*, Oxford: Oxford University Press.

Cignacco, E., Büchi, S. and Oggier, W. (2004) 'Hebammengeleitete Geburtshilfe in einem Schweizer Spital', *Pflege* 17(5): 253–61.

Cluett, E. and Bluff, R. (2003) *Principles and Practice of Midwifery Research*, London: Ballière Tindall.

Enkin, M. and Chalmers, I. (1982b) 'Effectiveness and satisfaction in antenatal care', in Enkin, M. and Chalmers, I. (eds) *Effectiveness and Satisfaction in Antenatal Care*, London: Heinemann Medical, pp. 266–90.

Farley, C.L. (2005) 'Midwifery's research heritage: a Delphi survey of midwife scholars', *Journal of Midwifery and Women's Health* 50(2): 122–8.

Iedema-Kuiper, H.R. (1996) *Geïntegreerde thuiszorg bij risico-zwangeren (Domiciliary risk in high risk pregnancies)*, doctoral thesis, Utrecht: Universiteit Utrecht.

Kirkham, M.J. (1989) 'Midwives and information-giving during labour', in Robinson, S. and Thomson, A.M. (eds) *Midwives, Research and Childbirth Vol 1*, London: Chapman and Hall, pp. 117–38.

Röckner, G., Wahlberg, V. and Ölund, A. (1989) 'Episiotomy and perineal trauma during childbirth', *Journal of Advanced Nursing* 14: 264–8.

Roumen, F.J.M.E. and Luyben, A.G. (1991) 'Safety of the term vaginal breech delivery', *European Journal of Obstetrics & Gynaecology and Reproductive Biology* 40(3): 171–7.

Schuster, U. (1998) 'Hebammengeburtshilfe: ein Projekt an der Universittsklinik Wien', *Oesterreichische Hebammenzeitung* 5: 152–3.

Simms, C., McHaffie, H., Renfrew, M. and Ashurst, H. (1994) *The Midwifery Research Database, MIRIAD: A sourcebook of information about research in midwifery*, Hale: Books for Midwives.

Sprung, G. (1998) 'Medikamentengabe während der Geburt. Ein Hebammenforschungsprojekt am KH Korneuburg', *Oesterreichische Hebammenzeitung* 6: 167–8.

Thomson, A.M. (1993) 'Pushing techniques in the second stage of labour', *Journal of Advanced Nursing* 18: 171–7.

Turnbull, D., Holmes, A. and Shields, N. *et al.* (1996) 'Randomised, controlled trial of efficacy of midwife-managed care', *Lancet* 348(9022): 213–18.

Van Lieburg, M.J. (1984) *C.G. Schrader's Memoryboeck van de vrouwens*, Amsterdam: Rodopi.

World Health Organisation (WHO) (1987) *Wenn ein Kind unterwegs ist . . . Bericht über eine Studie*, Oeffentliches Gesundheitswesen in Europa 26, Copenhagen: WHO Regional Office for Europe.

Chapter 10

The midwife historian

Lindsay Reid

'Never forget.' The teacher's words rang in my eleven-year-old ears. 'This – is history being made.' It was 1952. King George VI died that cold February day and there was a new young Queen. That was the first time that I realised that each one of us is a part of history and has a part to play in making history.

If history is common to us all, what makes a historian? And, more specifically, a midwife historian? This chapter will explore some aspects of this side of a midwifery career.

The scene is the sitting room of a flat belonging to Mary, a retired midwife. We have not met before and I am there in my role as midwife historian. We have introduced ourselves, had tea and chatted to break the ice. Now, the tape recorder is running and Mary (MM) is telling me (LR) about being a midwife in the 1940s and 1950s:

MM: (interrupting her train of thought) Are you a midwife yourself?
LR: Yes, I am . . .
MM: (significantly) Oh, well then . . . (carries on talking).

I was a Green Lady [Glasgow Municipal Midwife] for five years . . . it was just post-war and hospital beds weren't plentiful . . . worse than today. Someone would phone in to say that Mrs A or Mrs B was in labour and could she go into hospital?

If the answer was no, if there were no beds, we were sent out. Often you got a hostile reception . . . because a family was unprepared for this. They hadn't been prepared for a home confinement and they maybe had little in the way of bed-linen and towels and even the minimum of baby clothes . . . Many mothers were unbooked [with no antenatal care].

You had to palpate . . . make up your mind whether or not it was a spontaneous vertex presentation or a breech or whatever, check the foetal heart, the mother's blood pressure and the usual observations. At the same time you had to try and establish a reasonable relationship with the mother and the rest of the family. Usually when you went into the house it was full of neighbours or relations and you had to sort that out.

I'm talking about tenement houses in Glasgow, two apartments – a room and kitchen. They had box-beds. They would have had a sink but often no running hot water. Often you were dependent on boiling kettles or pots for hot water. Not many of them would have a bath in the house. As far as I recall they mostly had a toilet . . .

Usually the box-bed was in the kitchen and the heating was really a range in the kitchen. Because the mother was in labour and in these days it wasn't . . . the thing to have a husband present, husbands were shooed out the door. The family couldn't use the kitchen during this time.

The mother would have had the baby in the box-bed. Often in these circumstances, to avoid putting the baby into the bed with the mother, the handiest thing to put the baby in was a drawer. I got a reasonably sized drawer, emptied it, lined it with some sort of bedding and put the baby in.

[Some] women had booked and they were prepared. But some were unbooked . . . they usually borrowed bed-linen and towels from neighbours or extended family and Glasgow Corporation provided an initial layette for the baby.

I always worked on the principle that if you got a phone call you had to get your skates on because you couldn't depend on the husband's or the mother's report. The time that they would say, 'Oh it's all right', is the time when you would go in and discover the membranes had ruptured and the head was crowning. And the time that the husband would phone and say 'Oh the baby was imminent' is when the baby was born three days later. So you really had to . . . get your skates on and then make your own decisions.

We did breech deliveries at home. To my astonishment, on one of my refresher courses . . . I proceeded to deliver a breech until another midwife said to me, 'No you're not allowed to touch a breech. It's got to be the doctor.' That was in the mid-1970s . . . I think an experienced midwife is better than a first-time doctor delivering a breech.

LR: How did you handle it in a box-bed?
MM: With great difficulty. (Laughter) You'd practically to climb into the bed . . . The babies were all right . . . It was very satisfying.

(Reid 1997–2002: LR 27)

Personal midwifery

I was a latecomer to the profession of midwifery, although this was my goal from an early age. My history as a midwife moved through hands-on midwifery in maternity units and community, teaching and then research. Sometimes I held more than one post at a time, thereby widening my scope. For example, I was a midwife teacher and bank midwife at the same time; I was a research assistant and bank midwife together; and, for a time, I teamed being a midwife historian with a post in education and research at the RCM Scottish Board. In each area I wanted to change things – to change the way women were cared for, to give them choice without arguments, to remove the sometimes authoritarian role of the midwife (who at the same time was only obeying policies laid down for her) and to work more closely with women. Simultaneously, I felt the need for more autonomy for midwives – the need for midwives to have freedom to practise and take responsibility for their practice.

Becoming a midwife historian

In 1995, I became Research Assistant (RA) in midwifery for the RCM and the University of Glasgow. Initially, we were researching *Midwives and Woman-centred Care* (Hillan *et al.* 1997).

As RA, I had to do a literature search to give background and depth to the research. Two immediate questions emerged: what has happened in midwifery in Scotland before? And, where is the literature pertaining to our midwifery past?

I found that there was little written about midwifery in Scotland. Although midwifery history in England and Wales and internationally had attracted a number of authors, little had been written about Scottish midwifery and its history. A personal interest in the history of my country became more specific as I tried to find out about Scottish midwifery history. For instance, regulation of midwives came to England and Wales in 1902, but Scottish midwives had to wait until 1915 for the Midwives (Scotland) Act. Why was there this difference? What happened in the intervening years? What happened next? (Mander and Reid 2002). These questions threatened to overtake my current research and I resolved to find out the answers. However, although it was frustrating, my morphing into midwife historian had to wait until the completion of the current piece of research.

Are historians born or do they develop? Perhaps, we could say, a bit of both; it is difficult to speak for others. However, there must be an interest, a spark that becomes a flame. An awareness, an asking of questions, a quickening curiosity in history, in what has happened in the past comes first, sometimes unremarked upon, but which, with nurturing, can become progressively deeper. It is easy to use the word 'passion', but some people do develop a passion for the past. The historian develops, the passion becomes more organised, the historian studies, becomes immersed in, writes about and sometimes teaches history.

The midwife historian's path is similar, but the general history field will narrow into an area of particular specific interest. So, for the purpose of this chapter, a midwife historian has such a particular, or passionate, interest in midwifery history that she or he may study, write about and/or teach it, often in addition to the day job. The midwife historian also has the added benefit of understanding practical midwifery and its particular terminology (the 'insider': see below). This informs progress during development into the midwife historian. In addition, there may also be a special interest in a particular aspect of midwifery past: a particular time period; sometimes a specific country; and, possibly, a specific area or institution.

Finding out

Reading and research

How do we find out about the profession of midwifery in the past? By exploring, researching and relating events and happenings to what has gone before. Sources and methods include: reading books and journals, obtaining information from another person's work and research; examination of archives; schools and universities. Informally, scraps of history can be picked up anywhere: family stories told round the dinner table, family scrapbooks and the media, for example newspapers, television, radio, films, magazines, journals, books, textbooks, historical fiction, biographies and the internet. One significant feature of history is that books and archives do not go out of date. Styles of writing change, and ways in which authors, speakers or journalists present an event may be different. Nevertheless, each is a part of the rich tapestry of the past. It is the historian's privilege to examine that tapestry as minutely as necessary.

Minutes of the then statutory body, the Central Midwives Board for Scotland (CMB 1916–83, National Archives of Scotland (NAS)) gave me an important initial focus. However, the minuted Board activities raised further questions. For instance, I wanted to know more about the CMB chairmen. Archival names and dates were interesting, but what were they *like*? I was reading an old book of my father's – not overtly to do with midwifery. Words jumped out:

> Sir John Halliday Croom . . . tall, slender, debonair, with a short well-trimmed beard . . . lectured in a swallow-tailed, silk-faced evening coat, worn over a fancy waistcoat, and well-creased cashmere trousers. This combination of garments looked unusual, especially when he raised his hand and exclaimed, 'Mark me, gentlemen, and mark me well. Orange paste for your nails, a clean shirt every day, a flower in your buttonhole, and your fortune's made.'
>
> (Sutherland 1934: 81)

Sir John Halliday Croom was Professor of Midwifery at the University of Edinburgh and first chairman of the CMB (1916–21). The 'thumb-nail' sketch above, accidentally found in an old, some would say unimportant book, gave personal detail that CMB minutes do not provide. On the other hand, exploration of the

CMB minutes revealed much about its organisation and attitude towards midwives, including, for many years, their low status.

It took until 1977 for a midwife, Sheelagh Bramley, finally to be elected to the Chair (CMB 1916–83). Margaret Kitson, midwife and CMB member recalled:

> [W]hen I joined the CMB [in 1972], I was considered to be very young and inexperienced . . . There was a rather patronising attitude . . . It was necessary to begin with, on the Board, just to sit down, be quiet and listen . . . the CMB was very, very medically dominated.

She also remembered how Mary Turner (Chair 1978–83) changed things:

> In the most professional . . . way, without being . . . confrontational but by being very positive and . . . stating her case very clearly, listening to argument, but . . . in a very gentle way, changing the whole atmosphere in the Board so that it became much more possible for people to express their views.
>
> (Reid 2003: 304, 182; 1997–2002: LR 120)

I spent many days in the NAS with CMB minutes and other relevant archives: reading, writing, thinking, making connections. This was the formal archival research: it became a framework upon which to add the colour and life of narratives.

These came from midwives themselves. I was interested in what midwives thought, how they worked, how they felt about being very closely supervised after regulation began. I wanted to find how it was for midwives to change from being an unregulated profession to one that was very strictly controlled. Did the CMB ideal differ from midwifery in the real world? I needed to find out more, to add life to my study, to find the narrative. I had to add another dimension to being a midwife historian. I had to speak to midwives to find out what really happened 'on the ground'. This involved listening to and recording the voices and stories of midwives.

Oral history

Oral history has considerable potential for the history of midwives and for the midwife historian's work (Reid 2003: 309). Oral history, now an accepted form of historical research, is used to obtain information where little documented evidence exists or where the documented evidence is one-sided or suspect. It also revises history by challenging an accepted, usually written, view of an issue. Mid-wives did not traditionally write down their experiences and there is much that remains unknown about past midwifery practice. It is relevant for current midwives to elicit what has gone before in this way, to expand their knowledge and enhance their practice (Hunter 1999). As the written archival sources for the history of midwifery in Scotland omit details of midwifery practice and the careers of midwives, it is appropriate, where possible, to use oral history to examine the work and career histories of midwives in the comparatively recent past.

Outcomes of interviews depend on circumstances (Reid 2003: 313) and also on how much the interviewer knows. The interviewer can be an 'outsider', a 'naive interviewer', ready to ask intelligent questions but not knowing about the subject. However, from this 'innocent standpoint', the outsider can obtain much information. Or the interviewer can be an 'insider', a 'native interviewer', who knows about the subject, is possibly in an easier position and may achieve perhaps better, but usually different results. There are a couple of pitfalls for the novice insider: he or she needs to set aside any preconceived ideas so that the interviewee feels uninhibited; also, the insider interviewer should be aware of the temptation to use up precious interviewing time 'talking shop'. On the other hand, an interviewee, knowing that the interviewer is an insider, may be more likely to respond openly (Stanton and Thompson 1999). This is what happened in the vignette at the beginning of this chapter. Mary acknowledged my 'insider' status and probably spoke more freely because of this. Thus, as midwife historian and using oral history as a method of finding information, it has been an advantage to be able to claim my 'insider status'. Mary, and others, showed me through their narratives what being a midwife was like through the twentieth century: how, although they were closely supervised and bound strictly by CMB rules, on the district, until the early 1950s, they enjoyed a measure of autonomy and decision making. This disappeared in the years after the Second World War and the implementation of the National Health Service Act in 1948 and subsequent hospitalisation and medicalisation of the maternity services (Reid 2003).

So, I have found that using more than one method of researching midwifery history in Scotland has helped to give a well-rounded picture of what it was like. In addition, to use oral history alongside archival sources has attracted significant interest from members of the midwifery profession.

Making connections

There may be some readers who have difficulty in seeing why history and, in this instance, midwifery history, is important. They may ask what the point of studying it is when there are so many more pressing, immediate things to do. But, consider: when we are driving, we say, 'Mirror, signal, manoeuvre' – in that order. So it is with history in relation to our lives and work. It is by looking into, and taking note of, the rear-view mirror of history that we are able to understand and cope as well as we can with the present and move forward into the future with confidence.

This became evident as I moved more deeply into midwife historian mode and homed in on exploring midwifery in the twentieth century. Two linked yet distinct areas of controversy that are relevant to midwifery practice today emerged clearly. I have been aware of them and have felt uncomfortable about them since becoming a midwife.

First, there was the medicalisation of childbirth. Van Teijlingen *et al.* link this with midwifery as 'medicalisation of childbirth and midwifery' and define the term as:

> the increasing tendency of women to prefer a hospital delivery to a home delivery, the increasing trend toward the use of technology and clinical intervention in childbirth, and the determination of medical practitioners to confine the role played by midwives in pregnancy and childbirth, if any, to a purely subordinate one.
>
> (van Teijlingen *et al.* 2000)

Second, there was the paradox of the midwife: approved by statute to practise autonomously, and yet bound by policies, protocols and rules that negated a midwife's freedom to practise and make decisions with and on behalf of a mother and her baby.

Thus, there is an association between the diminishing of midwifery as an autonomous profession in twentieth-century Britain and the development of more medical interventionist practices, and more pain relief in labour linked with more mothers having their babies in hospital (Tew 1995). With these changes, midwives in the late twentieth century had a continuing struggle to maintain a measure of independence and faced challenges as great as those at the beginning of the century (Robinson 1990).

I had been living the history since I became a midwife. This included being a part of the uncomfortable state of midwifery; probably even going along with it because, as one midwife said to me, 'I felt as if my hands were *tied*' (Reid 1997–2002: LR 120); being involved with the new 'direct-entry' midwifery courses in the early 1990s; watching and commiserating as students returned to the classroom, deflated with what they saw out in the world of the clinical area; rejoicing with the publication of the Government-led documents on improving maternity care in the four countries of the UK (DH 1993; SHHD 1993; NIDHSS 1994; Welsh Office 1996); and joining in with writing, talking and researching about recommendations for improvements in maternity care with the term 'woman-centred care' becoming a focal point.

Now, plans for progress in maternity care that involve women as partners in their care and correspondingly higher levels of midwifery autonomy and freedom to practise are under way in countries all over the world (Reid 2007). These initiatives and many more are midwifery history being made. They are all informed by what has gone before.

Opportunities

Being a midwife historian creates opportunities. Some of these are obvious, such as searching the archives, libraries and the internet, making contact with knowledgeable scholars and historians, talking to groups in universities, conferences and church halls, and participating in workshops and seminars. A huge privilege is the chance to speak to midwives, sometimes very elderly, sometimes newly retired, sometimes still in practice, many in their own homes, about a subject that I, and they, hold dear. The importance of finding midwives who could tell me what it was like, give me stories and information that will be lost if they are not recorded, written down, disseminated, kept for future generations, cannot be overestimated. Midwives whom I have interviewed have invariably been supportive and enthusiastic. As we climbed the stairs to one elderly midwife's flat, she said 'This is a very exciting day for me.' This was not because she was going to see me. Rather, through this oral history interview she was going to be able to tell her story. She recognised her part in history and was glad to have this acknowledged.

Less obviously, being a midwife historian has offered me the opportunity to slow the tempo, look at the detail, check information, and tell myself, 'you are not in a hurry'. But surely this links with the pattern of best practice in normal midwifery. Think of translating this opportunity into midwifery clinical practice. Best practice does not include a need to see a target number of women in the antenatal clinic, an anxious surveillance over a clock-timed labour or a rush round the community in order to achieve as many postnatal visits as possible in a given time. An opinion from the 1920s said, 'You see, they [midwives] didn't do much – nature did it. A lot of midwifery is just waiting' (Reid 1997–2002: LR 61). Perhaps that elderly interviewee had a point. There's a lot to be said for knowledgeable watching and waiting.

Conclusion

We all need to be aware of our history. We could, and some do, function with knowledge of the present only. Yet, practice is more complete if we have knowledge of the past to inform the present and help to prepare for the future.

Nothing stands still. This struck me again as I thought about my career pathway to being a midwife historian. The benefit of my being a midwife, an 'insider', allowed Mary and other midwives to speak more freely midwife to midwife. This in turn widened my knowledge. I became more and more aware of the midwifery past: the CMB and its attitude to midwives; changes in practice through major events; and the need for positive change for childbearing women and midwives. I also was a part of midwifery change as it happened. This too, is now history. But change continues, and today's change will signpost tomorrow's history.

Commentary

Lindsay's paper provides us with a delightfully clear picture of what it means to be a midwife historian and, probably more importantly, why it matters. Her words bring to life the experience of the woman giving birth in what I knew as a 'single end' in Glasgow. She also breathes life into the characters for whom midwifery was a way of life. But it seems to have been a very different way of life from midwifery as we now know it.

On the other hand, some of what Lindsay's informants say is familiar: 'They didn't do much – nature did it.' This resonates very clearly with the very sensible advice that Nicky Leap offers to midwives: 'the less we do the more we give' (2000: 1).

Is it possible that there may be an element in midwifery of 'What goes around comes around'? Attention to history encourages us to contemplate the big picture, rather than keeping our eyes down, firmly fixed on the minutiae of practice or teaching or whatever our current focus happens to be. As well as providing the context, as Lindsay does so admirably, this big picture helps to put into proportion the challenges facing us. The big picture also lends to our impressions depth as well as breadth, allowing us to question what we do from a whole new perspective.

Lindsay introduces us to the generations of midwives of which we are a part. Although she refers particularly to the future generations, to whom the midwife historian has such a responsibility, we may think also of the past generations. I remember them well. Although at the time I may have dismissed them as 'dry old sticks', by reading their words, as reported by Lindsay, I am reminded of the glint in their eyes and the fervour they brought to all that they did. Thus, in the same way that they encouraged me to persevere in all that I did, I hope that I support those who are entering and making their way into and through midwifery.

The thought of the past leads to some reflection of how practice and other aspects of midwifery have changed and are changing. Knowing how we view the behaviour and words of previous generations leads to countless questions. One of the less comfortable questions relates to how future generations will look back at childbearing in the new millennium – the 'noughties'? Will my personal discomfiture, when I reflect on routine interventions and less than educational education, be mirrored in the reflections of future generations of midwives? Is it possible that the development of midwifery history will encourage the midwife of the future to reflect and act? Hopefully, such action on reflection will lead to healthier and happier outcomes for women and their babies and, of course, for midwives.

References

Central Midwives Board for Scotland (CMB) (1916–03) Minutes of Meetings, 16 February 1916–30 June 1983, NAS, CMB 1/1–9, Edinburgh: NAS, West Search Room, Charlotte Square.

Department of Health (DH) (1993) *Changing Childbirth, Part 1: Report of the expert maternity group*, London: HMSO.

Hillan, E., McGuire, M. and Reid, L. (1997) *Midwives and Woman-centred Care*, Glasgow: University of Glasgow and Royal College of Midwives, Scottish Board.

Hunter, B. (1999) 'Oral history and research Part 1: uses and implications', *British Journal of Midwifery* 7, July: 426.

Leap, N. (2000) 'The less we do the more we give', in Kirkham, M. (ed.) *The Midwife–Mother Relationship*, London: Macmillan, pp. 1–18.

Mander, R. and Reid, L .(2002) 'Midwifery power', in Mander, R. and Fleming, V. (eds) *Failure to Progress: The contraction of the midwifery profession*, London: Routledge, pp. 1–19.

Northern Ireland DHSS (NIDHSS) Maternity Unit Study Group (1994) *Delivering Choice: Midwife and GP-led maternity units*, Belfast: NIDHSS.

Reid, L. (1997–2002) Oral testimonies, cited as LR 1–128.

Reid, L. (2003) 'Scottish midwives: the Central Midwives Board for Scotland and practising midwives', unpublished Ph.D. thesis, University of Glasgow.

Reid, L. (2007) *Freedom to Practise*, London: Routledge.

Robinson, S. (1990) 'Maintaining the independence of the midwifery profession: a continuing struggle', in Garcia, J., Kilpatrick, R. and Richards, M. (eds) *The Politics of Maternity Care*, Oxford: Clarendon Press, pp. 61–91.

Scottish Home and Health Department (SHHD (1993) *Provision of Maternity Services in Scotland: A policy review*, Edinburgh: HMSO.

Stanton, J. and Thompson, P. (1999) Teaching session: 'Oral history and the history of medicine', in the course: 'Oral history and the history of medicine', Oxford, 18–22 October.

Sutherland, H. (1934) *A Time to Keep*, London: Geoffrey Bles.

Tew, M. (1995) *Safer Childbirth? A critical history of maternity care*, 2nd edition, London: Chapman and Hall.

van Teijlingen, E., Lowis, G., McCaffery, P. and Porter, M. (eds) (2000) *Midwifery and the Medicalization of Childbirth: Comparative perspectives*, Commack, NJ: Nova Science Publishers.

Welsh Office (1996) *Welsh Maternity Services Review: Maternal and early child health*, Cardiff: The Welsh Office.

Chapter 11

The global midwife

Valerie Fleming

As a child, one of the highlights of my holidays was to be taken to the local airport during the busy summer holiday weekend. From the observation area my brother and I scanned the skies to watch the planes coming in and I fantasised about where they were coming from and what sort of people would go on them. Certainly no one in my circle would ever have such opportunities! Several years later, as I worked as a bus conductress to supplement my student income, I was put on the route that went past the airport. Approximately once per hour we stopped right in front of the terminal building and, at some point during that year, I vowed I would get on a plane. That opportunity arose just after I had completed my midwifery training, whereupon I embarked on a rail tour round Europe for my holidays. The only possible way I could cram it all in and be back in time for night duty was to fly from London to Aberdeen. Despite that flight living up to all my expectations, I little believed that six months later I would be embarking on a global career, which has now spanned several decades. As I write this chapter, I am sitting on a plane somewhere over Europe, a now almost weekly part of my life.

As with all the other career paths outlined in this book, becoming a 'global midwife' is a combination of a desire to do the job, achieving the right qualifications, experience and expertise and working to achieve the goals, coupled with being in the right place at the right time. It is my intention to outline in this chapter the possibilities that exist for midwives to take a global role and how they may go about achieving this. I intend to use my own experiences and those of other midwives, some of whom I encounter in a variety of places, as illustrations.

Becoming a midwife

Despite a common definition of the midwife agreed upon by major bodies such as the WHO, the ICM and the International Federation of Gynecology and Obstetrics (FIGO) (WHO/ICM/FIGO 2005), there are numerous programmes leading to qualification as a midwife. For example, in the UK one becomes a midwife only in a university, either through a three-year programme or, for those who have previously qualified as nurses, a programme of 18 months. This is in complete contrast to Germany, where there is no university education for midwives and the three-year programme is undertaken in a vocational secondary school. Further afield, in countries such as India and South Africa, students complete programmes of four academic years at university to become nurse-midwives and, in Jordan, the programme consists of one year in a military hospital on completion of a nursing programme. Already difficulties can be seen in the recognition of qualifications. How can a midwife with a six-month obstetric placement as part of a nursing programme possibly be equivalent to one with a three-year bachelor's degree focused entirely on midwifery?

It is therefore absolutely vital, for anyone entering midwifery with a view to travelling, that they ensure that their qualification will be recognised in the country in which they want to work. This hit home to me when I had almost completed my nursing programme and the senior tutor came into our class saying that a new Common Market (as the European Union (EU) was then) regulation had been passed stating that nurses in one EU country could now work in any other provided that they had done geriatrics. As this was not part of our curriculum, she wanted to know if any of us were interested in an elective placement there. While I was not aware of it at the time, that was Directive 77/453/EEC (EEC 1977) and a similar one was passed for midwifery three years later – 80/154/EEC (EEC 1980a). Midwifery went even further with another Directive specifying minimum standards (EEC 1980b). Each of these regulations has been amended on several occasions, the latest being 2005/36/EC (EU 2005), at which time all health professions were brought together under the one regulation. The midwifery specifications, however, still incorporate the minimum standards. Indeed, if any nurse thinking of becoming a midwife through a programme in the UK with the purpose of working in mainland Europe is reading this chapter, he or she would be advised to read this Directive, as the UK qualification falls short of the minimum requirements and a period of consolidation is required. Although in 1977 I did not consciously harbour notions of working in another European country, I chose to do the geriatric placement, thereby gaining a really valuable experience in basic nursing.

Now, in the UK, things are very different. Not only are we governed by the EU regulations that inform those of our own NMC, but since our education takes place in universities, we also have to consider the Declaration of Bologna (1999). In this, ministers of 29 countries agreed to comparable university degrees, thus creating opportunities for university-educated midwives to advance their education in other signatory countries (now numbering 46). The countries that are signatories to this declaration vastly outnumber those of the EU, so ultimately this means that academic qualifications must be recognised in the signatory countries, while potentially professional qualifications are not. For the midwife wanting to work in one of the 15 countries this affects, this may well mean much negotiation.

Potential for midwives early in their careers

Although the midwifery regulations were passed just after I had completed my education, these were never alluded to either during or after I had completed the programme. One thing that was certain, however, after my first experience of European travel and flying, was that I wanted to travel. A few opportunities presented themselves through advertisements in professional journals, but all of them required considerably more experience than I had. Other options were with voluntary groups, such as Voluntary Service Overseas (VSO), but many of these were, and still are, for two-year periods, often in uncomfortable settings. At that stage, I was not convinced it was for me, but there are many midwives, whom I have subsequently met, who have found such experiences immensely valuable and have built their entire careers working in similar organisations.

My own plans were made together with an Australian midwife with whom I shared a flat. We planned an ambitious trip through western Asia to India and southeast Asia, ending up at my friend's home. Thereafter, I would fly back and fulfil my ambition to become a ward sister. However, it very quickly became evident that money was an obstacle and, to do this dream trip, I would have to work for an agency on my days off and find employment in Australia before returning. Sadly, at that time, Australia was only issuing one-year visas with no guarantee of renewal, so I opted instead for New Zealand, which wanted midwives (but not nurses) and was prepared to offer me permanent residence. While I have glossed over this issue in one sentence, it is important to say that, for anyone in the same position now, this did not happen easily. It is perhaps easier now, since the advent of the internet, but it is still time-consuming and bureaucratic. Negotiations must be made with prospective employers, consulates and midwifery regulatory bodies. Clearly, where regulatory bodies exist, potential global midwives must check with them that their qualifications will be recognised or, if not, if the requirements are acceptable. Often requirements involve a period of continuing education for which a fee is charged and during which the midwife cannot practise. In turn, this may make immigration difficult, as a job offer will not be made until the qualification is obtained. While this may appear to be a vicious circle, it is usually possible through sharing all the correspondence with each of the parties concerned to reach a compromise. However, the fundamental driver will always be the labour market at the time, and such was the case in 1980 when my friend and I finally made some of our epic journey though Asia.

Wars and invasions meant that our plans to travel through western Asia had to be abandoned and, instead, we flew to India to begin a three-month exploration of the subcontinent. I was affected greatly by the poverty, masses of people and the bureaucracy there and, after two weeks, desperately wanted to escape. However, I persisted and eventually in my travels reached Tiruneveli in Tamil Nadu, where I had been in contact already with a doctor known to one of my colleagues in Aberdeen. When we met her she was delighted that two midwives had come to see her and took us to the hospital where she worked. On the door were the mortality statistics for the month and, to someone who had only ever seen one maternal death, they were frightening, while to this doctor they were a vast improvement. She felt that they could be much better if there were sufficient midwives to work there. Naturally we volunteered and suddenly we were there, earning no money but a wealth of experience. We were not registered with the Indian Nursing Council, but such was the need that this was irrelevant to the local authorities. The labour market had dictated what was required and we were in the right place.

The same was said for my next placement on the Thai–Kampuchean border. Civil war had broken out in Cambodia and refugees were flooding over the border into Thailand in the hope of escaping persecution. Infectious diseases such as cholera and typhoid were endemic and, as I was nearby and had been vaccinated, I felt I could be of some use. The International Red Cross was delighted to see me and, once more, I felt able to be of use while building up my own experience.

It was therefore as a much more experienced midwife than I had anticipated that I finally arrived in New Zealand, where I mixed with a large group of international midwives, most of whom had come on one-year working visas. I was delighted to have my permanent residency, however, as I stayed in New Zealand for 16 years, pursuing a more recognisable career working as a midwife in various settings. Two exemplars stand out, however, that have relevance for the aspiring global midwife of today. Four years after I had arrived in New Zealand, I decided on a trip back to the UK to visit family. At that point I discovered that permanent residence was only permanent as long as I stayed in the country. The authorities no longer had any need of midwives, so residence would not be renewed. My solution was to apply for (and gain) citizenship. Dual nationality in my career today is extremely useful!

The second example was my own drive to improve my education. New Zealand offered opportunities that the UK did not and I pursued first an Advanced Diploma of Midwifery and then a bachelor's degree by distance learning. With the Declaration of Bologna and other systems in place for recognition of prior learning in many countries, for midwives to gain a bachelor's degree is relatively straightforward and may involve as little as one semester's full-time study. However, in the 1980s it involved four years of full-time equivalent study to gain those two qualifications. What they did was make me want to learn more and, before leaving New Zealand, I had gained my D.Phil., had a good career record, had learned a lot about international health, in particular women's health, and had the confidence to apply for a position in what the advert called a 'World Health

Organisation Collaborating Centre'. I was successful in attaining that position and the last 13 years have been spent as an academic midwife pursuing an international career.

Global opportunities

There are perhaps more opportunities for midwives to pursue international careers now than ever before. Prevailing health problems that continue to face many regions include the increasing gap between the health of the rich and poor and unacceptable mortality/morbidity statistics. In addition, there is a resurgence of many infectious diseases, for example tuberculosis, meningitis and hepatitis, as well as sexually transmissable diseases, such as HIV/Aids, and their associated problems. Many countries and communities are faced with women with lifestyle-related problems, such as unhealthy diets, too little exercise, smoking and alcohol and substance misuse. Increasing numbers of some populations suffer from stress, mental ill health and other chronic diseases, while others face the effects of poverty and unemployment (Fleming and Holmes 2005). The opportunities are thus plentiful for both midwives with little experience and those with many years of working at senior levels. Both have valuable contributions to make and positions can be short or long term, paid or voluntary. For the remainder of this chapter I intend to outline some of these possibilities.

Crisis situations

In the various news media, we are faced almost daily with stories of natural disasters and civil wars. While the plea is often for money or equipment, there is always a need for human resources and midwives are particularly valuable, as many populations include young women who often have been violently sexually abused. Women, too, are frequently considered of lesser importance than men or children and their health needs do not receive priority assistance locally in times of crisis. The voluntary aid organisations are among those that do their best to fill these gaps. Some of these are faith-based, while others are secular in their orientation; midwives aspiring to work with such organisations need to recognise this to ensure that their own beliefs do not clash with those of the organisation with which they propose to work.

Any midwife planning to work in crisis situations needs to have not only the professional and technical skills to carry out the job, but also needs to be strongly aware of local cultural beliefs and values in order to embrace these or, at the very least, not cause offence with certain practices. Perhaps one of the strongest examples of this is the practice of female genital mutilation (FGM), which takes place in many parts of Africa. Girls, either shortly after birth or any time until they reach puberty, have their external genitalia excised to varying degrees, the stated aim being to keep them celibate in preparation for marriage. When sexual intercourse does take place it is usually extremely painful for the woman and often leads to chronic urinary and genital infections. When the woman with a more radical form of FGM gives birth, it is necessary to reverse this mutilation in order for the baby to be born safely. After the birth, the woman or her husband frequently requests that she is returned to her pre-birth state.

While most western countries have outlawed such a practice, it remains the norm for many women in some of the countries in which midwives will work. Midwives going to work in times of crisis in such areas need to be aware of this, and other similar practices, and deal only with the crisis, while remembering that many international organisations are working together with concerned local groups and individuals in an attempt to change such practices.

Midwives working in crisis situations are generally responding to some specific emergency and will find themselves working and living in horrific conditions. It is essential to be aware of this before agreeing to embark upon such work as, once in the affected area, there is generally little chance to opt out and return home. However, the rewards of such work are substantial, not only through the immediate help that can be given to women and their families, but also by working in the multidisciplinary teams that are the norm at such times. The benefits of working in such teams include the sharing of knowledge and experience, as well as the making of lasting friendships and finding out about where the next job opportunity might be.

Indeed, midwives, and of course others, choosing to work in crisis situations would not be doing their jobs properly if their postings were long term. To work in a crisis situation means to go in as part of a rescue effort and deliver the appropriate package. As mentioned above, there are many crisis situations in the world, and it is often the same group of people who move from one to the next, thereby building up a body of experience and expertise that is immediately transferable.

Although I have talked about the voluntary aid organisations in this section, it does not always mean that a midwife's work in crisis situations is unpaid. Indeed, in some instances a highly attractive salary may be offered. As with any other position, it is vital to ensure well in advance what the terms and conditions of employment are to facilitate informed choice.

Reconstruction

While responding to crisis situations is something that happens rapidly, reconstruction usually comes about following much negotiation with governments and large organisations, which are often, although not exclusively, agencies of the United Nations (UN), such as the WHO. Other major stakeholders in reconstruction work are frequently international banks, such as the World or Asian Development Banks, while yet others are individual governments of wealthier countries or foundations launched by philanthropists, such as the Aga Khan Foundation, while several faith-based organisations contribute. To the outsider, reconstruction work may often appear to be fragmented and lacking in coordination, resulting in duplication of effort. Indeed, this was an issue raised frequently by respondents worldwide to the UK's Department for International Development research consultation (DFID 2008).

Often, reconstruction work lasts for several years and is based on promoting public health or, more recently and more specifically, achieving the Millennium Development Goals (UN 2000). Stakeholders committed themselves to achieving these eight goals by 2015 and many countries in the world, most noticeably in the Far East, have made enormous strides and expect to achieve all the goals on target. For other countries, the outlook is not so positive and, at the midterm evaluation (UN 2007), several countries advised that at least one (and in some cases several) more of the goals would not be achievable by 2015 unless huge amounts of international aid were given. Three of the goals are directly concerned with women's health: these being numbers 3 to 5:

3   promote gender equality and empower women;
4   reduce child mortality;
5   improve maternal health.

Sadly, out of the eight goals, that which is least likely to be achieved is goal number 5. In most cases, this is due to a lack of skilled birth attendants to provide adequate antenatal care, so midwives can make a vast difference by working for both large and small organisations to help improve the dreadful birth statistics that still dominate some parts of the world. For example, the extremes of maternal mortality ratios (UN 2007) stand at 2,100/100,000 in Sierra Leone, compared with 1/100,000 Ireland. In developing countries generally, the figures are 450/100,000 in comparison with 9/100,000 in developed countries. In Europe we cannot afford to be complacent as, while the Irish statistics are exemplary, in the Commonwealth of Independent States (CIS, former Soviet Union countries) the maternal mortality rate is still 51/100,000.

Working with statistics such as these can be a daunting task and midwives need to choose carefully the type of work to which they feel the most suited. In some of the smaller organisations, for example, a midwife might find him- or herself the only 'international' at a remote field station with very little equipment. While this may be very daunting and lonely, it provides an opportunity for midwives to exercise all their clinical skills, often in very difficult situations. Many women or their families will not seek professional assistance until they have exhausted all the other possibilities and, if they do approach the foreign midwife, it is often with suspicion. Care therefore needs to be taken by midwives when posted to remote field stations to ensure that they become fully conversant with local beliefs and practices and do not immediately set out to contradict these. As shown earlier in this chapter, FGM is commonplace in parts of Africa with latest UN statistics (2007) showing that 97.5 per cent of women are subjected to some degree of this practice. The midwife who is working in a long-term capacity is ideally placed to begin re-education of women in this situation, working slowly with local people of influence to build up trust and acceptance and by being willing to listen and in turn learn from local culture.

Rather than being entirely on their own, however, midwives working for small organisations may often find themselves lodging with other professionals (often engineers) working for the same or other organisations. This makes them part of a small community, not only sharing accommodation but also aspirations and ideals. A close-knit community such as this is almost like a family – accompanied by its own highs and lows.

Finding such positions usually comes by word of mouth and, as mentioned earlier; often the same group of people may be seen moving from project to project. That can only happen once a midwife has become established and is known to be capable of producing good results. The reverse may happen, where a midwife who has not been successful is unable to find other similar employment. To enter such positions for the first time often means a good deal of determination and patience, as vacancies are frequently not advertised. If midwives simply want the experience of working for such organisations and do not mind which, they have more scope. They still need to trawl through many websites and write to numerous people. If they feel more restricted, for example in terms of working with religious organisations or those with a particular philosophy, they will have less searching to do but less potential.

Working for some of the larger organisations, such as the UN's various agencies, offers different possibilities. Applications are made via a standard competitive process. Qualifications such as master's degrees are often sought. However, such agencies may offer the possibility of internships during master's degrees to raise awareness of the agencies and the type of work that they offer. These are generally unpaid positions, but the intern will be attached to a specific programme and may get the chance to visit the areas where the project is taking place. For example, in 2007, when I was working with the WHO on a project, a regional meeting was held in Zambia. All the interns working for the project were included in that meeting, thereby gaining first-hand experience of working at a strategic level within this large organisation.

Midwives may be employed by these agencies for specific projects that are likely to be based in their headquarters or in the various regional offices. Country offices nearly always employ local people, though 'internationals' may be seconded for varying periods of time. The specific project for which a midwife will be employed will reflect not only skills as a midwife but the education and experience she or he has subsequently received. For example, an initiative known as 'Making Pregnancy Safer' is supported by several agencies and midwives employed on that project may be employees of any of the organisations involved but is most likely to be required to be an expert in education, international health or in leading teams of people. Working for such large organisations, particularly at the level of individual projects, nearly always involves temporary contracts but, as with the smaller organisations, there are generally opportunities to move from project to project depending on the strength of experience, expertise and track record.

Another way in which midwives can become involved with the work of large organisations is not to work for them but to work with them. Most of my own recent experience has been in this area, so I intend to finish this chapter in the way in which I started it; that is, by outlining some of the recent projects I have run in recent years and showing how I managed to win the tenders for these projects and carry them out.

As indicated earlier in the chapter, I chose to join a university department that was a WHO Collaborating Centre (WHOCC). I had little real sense of what this meant, but quickly made it my business to find out. I made sure that the Centre's director was aware of work I had done and where I felt I could be useful. I was privileged to be invited to the biennial meeting of the Global Network of Collaborating Centres, where I was able to see the group in action and establish contacts with those people who shared my interests in women's health. During this time, I was continuing to develop my profile as an academic and improve my foreign language skills. In turn, this led me to other international meetings, where I continued to build up a network of contacts, thereby securing a secondment to a German university for a semester as a visiting professor. In turn, this led to more contacts, two of whom are currently working with me on another project funded by the EU.

Another important contact was a nurse from Jordan who was Dean of an academic faculty and was keen to establish academic midwifery in her country. Much email discussion followed and, some two years later, we were awarded a grant from the British Council for four years to develop a programme, the graduates of which are now studying for doctoral degrees in the UK and elsewhere. Through management of the programme, I was invited in 2007 to run a pre-doctoral programme for a group of Palestinian nurses and midwives with master's degrees. This programme was jointly sponsored by the WHO, an Israeli university, an external agency and my own institution.

As a direct result of our WHOCC status, I (by this stage the Centre's deputy director) was invited to tender along with all the other WHOCCs in Europe to do a scoping study on reconstructing midwifery and nursing education in post-war Kosovo. We won this tender and, after carrying out the work, were invited to implement it. This was a much harder task, but provided experience for many of my colleagues and those from other institutions who had not previously had such opportunities. All of them spent from one to six months in Kosovo working with locals, while I commuted, spending one week per month there. It was a proud moment when, after three difficult years, our first graduates received their degrees.

I have carried out a number of other consultancies for WHO and other organisations, during which I come across other consultants. Some of these are freelance and others employees. In both the education and clinical fields, I believe that freelance consultants have a career lifespan of approximately two years (though others would dispute this), as ideas are changing so rapidly that knowledge quickly becomes outdated. Midwives need to decide how they are going to stay in touch with these changes if they are going to freelance long term. Additionally, midwives spending any length of time in countries other than their own need to decide whether they are going to be part of the international community, or whether to spend more time with locals. During my time in Kosovo, as with other projects, I made many friends, mostly from among the Kosovars; but there was also a thriving British community that had activities of its own as well as its own favourite haunts for nightlife!

Conclusion

In this chapter, I have shown many of my own experiences in order to illustrate the rich tapestry of opportunities available to midwives seeking to become global in their own approach to their work. Both the projects I have mentioned above and the many consultancies I have run for the WHO have involved an incredible amount of hard work; indeed shift work did not end when I moved into academic life! There are also many disappointments, as much work gets invested in preparing research proposals or tenders for funding only to be rejected by those with the money. At times, when waiting in an uncomfortable airport for six hours in the middle of the night, I question myself. However, it is extremely rewarding work and begets ever more work.

Commentary

Valerie's account provides a vivid picture of a midwifery role that is very different from the one we usually envisage. Her writing creates an impression of a 'can do' approach, for which we lesser mortals are full of awe. Her penultimate sentence, though, shows us that such jet-setting may be something other than just high flying!

As well as the good news, Valerie provides priceless insights into the reality of working in less than familiar settings. Her harrowing account of the widespread practice of what she terms 'female genital mutilation' (FGM) brings home the sensitivity of practising in an unfamiliar location. The midwife working in the UK is likely occasionally to attend a woman who has been subjected to this form of abuse (Sosa 2004). The UK midwife's position is very different from that of the midwife, described by Valerie, who is endeavouring to provide care in a developing country.

The sensitivity of such situations will only serve to make midwives' practice even more challenging. They will also require a high level of political skills; by political, I mean in the sense of the dictionary definition of 'astutely contriving'. It may be that Politics with a capital 'P' will also feature in other aspects of the global midwife's work. This possibility may be gleaned from Valerie's mention of some of the countries to which she travels and the international organisations with whom she works.

Thus, political skills and supreme sensitivity are the qualifications needed for the global midwife. Such skills and sensitivity are essential to allow effective decisions to be made in 'prickly' situations. This applies particularly to situations involving cultural practices that we ordinarily find abhorrent, or when working with countries or agencies whose regimes are antithetical to our own principles.

Thus, it is apparent that global midwives, perhaps like their more earth-bound co-professionals, need to have a very clear vision of their personal objectives. This vision will help these midwives to address the priorities that are important to them and the women with whom they work. Identifying such priorities will help them to address the crucial needs of the women and their babies, while other levels and agencies focus on the less manageable factors.

References

Declaration of Bologna (1999) *Joint Declaration of European Ministers of Education*, 19 June.

Department for International Development (DFID) (2008) *Research Strategy 2008–13*, London: Crown Copyright.

European Economic Community (EEC) (1977) *Directive Concerning Mutual Recognition of Nursing Qualifications*, Directive 77/453/EEC, Brussels: EEC.

European Economic Community (EEC) (1980a) *Directive Concerning Mutual Recognition of Midwifery Qualifications*, Directive 80/154/EEC, Brussels: EEC.

European Economic Community (EEC) (1980b) *Directive Defining Minimum Standards in Midwifery Education*, . . ., Directive 80/155/EEC, Brussels: EEC.

European Union (EU) (2005) *Directive Concerning Mutual Recognition of Health Service Professionals' Education*, Directive 2005/36/EC, Brussels: EU.

Fleming, V. and Holmes, A. (2005) *Basic Nursing and Midwifery Education in Europe*, Copenhagen: WHO.

Sosa, G. (2004) 'The African Well Women Clinic at the Whittington Hospital NHS Trust', *MIDIRS Midwifery Digest* 14(2): 255–60.

United Nations (UN) (2000) *Millennium Development Goals*, Geneva: UN.

United Nations (UN) (2007) *Millennium Development Goals Mid-term Review*, Geneva: UN.

World Health Organisation (WHO) (2005) *Maternal Mortality in 2005: Estimates developed by WHO, UNICEF, UNFPA, and the World Bank*, Geneva: WHO.

World Health Organisation/International Confederation of Midwives/ International Federation of Gynecology and Obstetrics (WHO/ICM/ FIGO) (2005) *Definition of the Midwife*, Geneva: WHO.

Chapter 12

The independent midwife

Nessa McHugh

7a.m.: I am on my way to visit Beth; her partner, Andy, has phoned to say that Beth's labour has built up and she would now like me to visit. Having spoken to Beth, I think she is right. I have already contacted Allison, my midwifery partner, to let her know what is happening, so that she can plan her day and get her children off to school.

7.40 a.m.: I arrive at Beth's house; the last couple of miles are up a farm track and, as I get out of the car, I can see right across the valley – it is a beautiful morning. When I go in to see Beth, the lights are low and there is soft music playing in the background. Beth looks like she is labouring well and Andy is massaging her, whispering encouragement as another contraction washes over her. Quickly and quietly I bring my birth kit into the house and get everything I need organised, being careful not to disturb Beth with my activity.

I contact Allison again to let her know that I think Beth appears to be in good labour.

8.00 a.m.: Beth is in the pool and I have written down my observations and plan of action. As labour intensifies, Andy and Beth's sister, Sarah, are with Beth, supporting her through each contraction. I stay in the background, observing and waiting until I am needed.

8.15 a.m.: Beth starts the deep groaning of all women who are getting ready to give birth. There is a subtle shift in the atmosphere, Beth now holding on to her sister as she breathes through the contractions. Allison silently appears in the room. We make eye contact but say nothing.

8.20 a.m.: Beth leans forward in the pool and I look into the eyes of her baby as her head emerges into the water. I can hear Andy telling Beth he can see the baby. At the next contraction, Beth gives a small grunt and her baby slithers out. She reaches down to greet her new daughter, Ruby.

8.30 a.m.: As Ruby nuzzles Beth, the placenta has separated and is caught in a nearby bowl.

11 a.m.: Beth is lying on her bed with Ruby. Jamie, her little boy, has arrived with Grandma and is sitting on the bed inspecting his new sister.

Allison and I retreat to the kitchen to finish writing up our notes and to ensure that the family enjoys some privacy together.

It is a beautiful day to be born.

This chapter is an account of my experience of practising as an independent midwife. My practice enables me to choose to carry a small caseload of women and provide back-up for other midwives, while also continuing to work as a midwifery lecturer. The above vignette provides a snapshot of the intimacy of midwifery practice, where the midwife has had the time to get to know a woman and her family well throughout their work together. The vignette was written to encapsulate an experience of birth that, for me, is the essence of midwifery, namely the relationship between the woman and her midwife. This is something that I have experienced more as an independent midwife than in any other area of my midwifery career. In the vignette, I am in the background of the birth as it unfurls. The relationship that I had already built up with Beth enhanced my ability to assess her well-being and that of her baby. I believe that, with this relationship established, it becomes possible to observe and assess the progress of labour on many of the interconnected levels of human experience. I also believe that, when you get to know a woman and her family throughout her pregnancy, not only does this impact on how you relate to her in labour – it also serves to enhance the post-partum support you can provide. Independent Midwives UK (IM-UK) offers the following definition:

Independent Midwives are fully qualified midwives who, in order to practise the midwife's role to its fullest extent, have chosen to work outside the NHS in a self-employed capacity, although we support its aims and ideals. The midwife's role encompasses the care of women during pregnancy, birth and afterwards.

(IM-UK 2009)

Working independently presents both advantages and challenges for midwives, who will have worked within the NHS either as qualified midwives or as part of their midwifery education. At the time of writing, the majority of independent midwives work completely outside the NHS as most of us are now unable to secure honorary contracts of employment (although the situation does vary across Britain) and we are also unable to obtain professional indemnity insurance. This means that the majority of our clients will be booked for home births, or we will provide antenatal and postnatal midwifery care and act as a birthing partner if the birth is planned to take place in hospital.

At the time of writing, there are estimated to be fewer than 200 independent midwives in the UK, the majority of whom are members of IM-UK, which was formerly known as the Independent Midwives Association (IMA). All these midwives could probably give different reasons for practising independently, their motivation to work in this way and, probably, differing accounts of their practice experiences. Naturally, I can only write directly of my own experiences; however, it may be possible to suggest one shared factor among this very diverse group of midwives – namely, that they are passionate about the desire to establish their own ways of working with women. This passion is so strong that they are prepared to stand outside the NHS and wrestle with issues such as a lack of professional indemnity insurance in order to practise what I believe to be relational midwifery. Van der Hulst (1999) proposed that contemporary midwifery care is comprised of four distinct aspects; these are identified in Table 12.1.

Although van der Hulst identified the four aspects of midwifery work in relation to Dutch midwifery, it is clear that they can also be applied to midwifery in the UK and other settings. When I reflect on my working life as a midwife, I can see how these four aspects have been present in all the different midwifery settings in which I have worked. So far, my independent practice has been the only midwifery experience that has given me enough time and space

Table 12.1 Aspects of midwifery work (van der Hulst 1999)

Aspect	Description
Obstetric technical care	This relates to the observations, procedures and interventions that are undertaken to establish or ensure the well-being of the mother and baby.
Risk selection	In the majority of maternity care systems, women's care is based on a selection process that identifies the potential or actual risk status of the mother and baby. Risk selection involves the midwife using screening processes and then referring the woman on as deemed appropriate within the system the midwife is working in.
Social environment of the client	Here midwives tailor their working activities to take into account the psychosocial, emotional and spiritual needs of the women they work with. For this to work successfully, midwives need to move beyond a purely medicalised approach to care and view women as women with distinct individual needs.
Relational care	Good midwifery care depends upon the establishment of a trusting relationship between the woman and the midwife. The key elements of this relationship are based upon the recognition that it is an equal partnership based upon empowerment, openness and self-activation on behalf of both sides of the partnership.

to restore the balance between van der Hulst's four aspects within my clinical life. Like all midwives, I need good technical skills and the ability to assess well-being. However, when I work directly with women, rather than with an institution, these aspects harmonise with the considerations of the individual woman and the relationship of mutual trust that we aim to establish.

Being self-employed is one of the key aspects of independent practice that sets it apart from working for an employer such as the NHS. Working independently means you have a different relationship with your clients; one where the contract of employment is negotiated directly between the woman and the midwife. I would argue that the intimate nature of this working relationship is a result of the partnership it engenders. However, when the midwife is an employee of an institution, the ensuing relationship between a woman and her midwife is mediated by the midwife's contract to that institution and, therefore, by the nature of that institution and the complexity of the service that it endeavours to supply.

It can be argued that the common result of this relational triangle is an imbalance in what van der Hulst has identified as the main aspects of midwifery work. Reflecting on my own working experiences, I would suggest that van der Hulst's imbalance represents the challenges faced by midwives working in institutional settings, where there is arguably an emphasis on technical care and risk selection, to the potential detriment of those aspects concerned with relational care and the social environment of the client. Lawrence Beech and Phipps (2008) have proposed that, in our contemporary society, we do not fully recognise the significance and impact of birth on women's emotional well-being and the subsequent transition into motherhood. They go on to suggest that this lack of recognition is reflected within the systems that serve our birthing culture:

> It is generally expected that the woman should be satisfied with the birth of a live baby, irrespective of the way the birth happened. The failure to acknowledge and address the mother's experiences leaves too many women with traumatizing memories, rather than positive and empowering ones. Often this is because we have allowed systems to develop that interfere with the birth process.
>
> (Lawrence Beech and Phipps 2008: 69)

Independent practice has the potential to provide a way of practising midwifery that addresses some of the above issues. It has enabled me to keep practising midwifery in a way that allows a balance between the different aspects of my midwifery work.

A personal journey towards independence

I started in independent practice in 2004, having qualified as a midwife in 1990. When I made the decision to become a midwife in 1984, I quickly knew that I wanted to become an independent midwife. Then, as now, I believed in the principle of working with women directly, where equality and partnership are the bedrock of any professional relationship. Later on, as I gained experience of working as a midwife, I wanted to have more control of how I organised my working life. My perception of what independent practice entailed was rooted in my personal feminist philosophy. Kaufmann states that a feminist midwifery profession '[s]upports and values the women who work within it, asking them to work in solidarity with each other and with the women in their care in order to help all women have the birth experience they deserve' (2004: 9).

Looking back now, it seems hard to believe that my journey to independent midwifery practice took so long. I had aimed to start as soon as I could, but even the best laid plans don't always turn out the way you expect. In 1985, I took what was then the most readily available route to midwifery, training first as a nurse and then as a midwife. In 1994, having become frustrated at working in a system that made it difficult to work with women in the way that I wanted, I decided to set up as an independent midwife. I had already met independent midwives at national Association of Radical Midwives (ARM) meetings and I had attended workshops and study days to find out more about how midwives became independent and what the key issues were. I can remember wondering: Would I be able to earn enough money to replace my NHS wage?, Would there even be any clients in the area where I was based?, Would I be working in isolation?, How would I organise the services my prospective clients would need? Up to this point in my working life I was used to a regular income, and I worked in a large and complex organisation surrounded by other professionals who could clearly identify my role and where I fitted into the system.

Having found some answers to my questions, I started making my plans and was contacted by a couple of potential clients. However, my move towards self-employment and independent practice was dealt a severe blow when the RCM decided to withdraw professional indemnity insurance (PII) from independent midwives in 1994. Daunted by the prospect of working without affordable insurance (and even now that is unavailable), I gradually moved into teaching and reluctantly shelved my plans for independent practice.

Insurance considerations aside, the decision to become an independent midwife is hedged with many issues. Not least among these is the move from being an employee to becoming self-employed, or moving from student status, having trained within NHS institutions, to qualified status on the outside of those same institutions. Anxiety about being unable to earn a living can act as a deterrent to starting up in practice. Hobbs (1997) advised that, initially, midwives should consider how they plan to support themselves until they have clients booked. Starting up a practice involves not just establishing a client base, but also buying and maintaining equipment, and determining which are the best suppliers. Having a network of experienced independent midwives to call upon for information, support and advice was invaluable to me as I worked out what I needed and where to obtain it. Although there are only a few independent midwives in Scotland, I have never felt unsupported. My experiences have always been that other independent midwives are generous with their time, advice and support. I have found that the majority of independent midwives I have got to know over the years are very good at liaising both with each other and with other midwives and health professionals.

The concerns about insurance remain, especially in the current climate, in which the debates about professional risk and professional liability appear to have become blurred by issues occurring within less heavily regulated professions. Of all the health professions, midwifery remains the most heavily regulated. Each time I meet with prospective clients, we discuss in depth the issues of insurance, midwifery supervision and professional responsibility. Such discussions form the bedrock of any future working relationships and also reinforce my concept of what it means to be an autonomous practitioner.

Autonomous practice and client choice

Given that the NHS provides a complex maternity care system, it would not be unreasonable to wonder why women would chose to book with an independent midwife. After all, why pay for a service that is widely available free of charge? My experience of practising independently echoes that of many of my independent colleagues, in that women seek out an independent midwife because the service that they are looking for is not available to them in their local area. Frequently, women want continuity of midwife and to know the midwife who will be with them when they go into labour. Women will, therefore, choose an independent midwife because the alternative might be one midwife from a large team of midwives whom they may not have met before. The importance for women in labour of already knowing their midwife is often dismissed by sceptics, who claim that all women really want is someone who is skilled and kind. Pilley Edwards' (2000) study of women planning home births highlighted the importance of knowing and, therefore, being able to trust the midwife who was with you in labour. In the study, women reported fears about being transferred into hospital unnecessarily. For some women this fear was made worse by the fact that they did not really know their midwives. Where midwives had been able to provide continuity, women perceived their relationship as providing personal support and professional competencies. This blend of personal and professional was seen as crucial for mother–midwife interaction and achievable only when there was continuity in the interaction.

Women may also decide to book with an independent midwife if they experience difficulty in accessing specific sets of skills, such as vaginal breech birth, home VBAC (vaginal birth after Caesarean section), home birth or home water birth. From my own experiences, and from the experiences of independent midwifery colleagues, a significant number of women will seek out independent midwifery care because of their previous birth experiences and a subsequent desire to have more control over what will happen to them in their current pregnancy.

Independent practice is criticised for providing a limited and potentially elitist service, because women have to be able to pay for their midwifery care. There is arguably an element of truth in this accusation, as independent midwifery care is not free and, therefore, it is not equally available to all women. However, there is a broad spectrum of women who access independent midwives and many midwives try to adopt flexible systems of payment and barter. IM-UK has proposed a model of care, based on the original IMA NHS Community Midwifery Model, that would enable independent midwives to contract into local health care providers, such as Primary Care Trusts and Health Boards. The model of contracting in offers another route of midwifery care provision that would provide more women with potential choice of continuous care by a known midwife. Midwives offering this service would be contracted on a fee per client basis, in a manner similar to the way in which opticians and pharmacists are currently contracted.

Independent midwifery is one of a number of ways in which the autonomy of the midwife is clearly manifested. As autonomous practitioners, midwives can practise independently upon the point of qualifying and registration. This ability of midwives to establish a self-employed working practice could be cited as evidence of the autonomy of the midwifery profession. However, it is the very autonomy of independent midwives that can sometimes appear to place them at odds with the contemporary health environment. Working outside a clear management structure also places independent midwives in a potentially difficult position – how do you deal with or discipline a midwife who has no manager to report to?

It would appear that the answer to this would be to use midwifery supervision as a quasi-management tool and then report the midwife to the NMC. The NMC is the regulatory body for nursing and midwifery and, as such, has a responsibility for any disciplinary or investigatory procedures involving registrants. Being investigated by your professional body is a daunting prospect for any midwife, but for an independent midwife this can be particularly difficult. If you are suspended from practice pending investigation, you are effectively prevented from earning your living through midwifery. If there are no charges proved, it is virtually impossible to claim back any lost earnings. Wagner, writing about what he has termed a 'global witch hunt', states:

> It is no coincidence that 70% of the accused in my sample are midwives, all in independent practice where they are not under the immediate control of doctors. Fear of being investigated by authorities is a strong deterrent to independent midwives.
>
> (2004: 36)

Working independently can mean being perceived as an 'outsider'. Different hospitals have different ways of organising themselves and it can be challenging to negotiate systems that are not always apparent, especially if you cannot find the right person to provide support and information from within the system. As an outsider, it can be difficult communicating with other health professionals who may not understand alternative ways of working or who choose to display outward hostility towards either independent midwives or their clients. The following vignette relates to the transfer of a client, Jo, to hospital following a long labour, demonstrating the move from a holistic perspective of birth into a completely different setting. Jo was transferred from a setting corresponding to van der Hulst's concept of relational care into a setting that could be identified as having risk selection and obstetrical technical care dominating any other considerations.

The decision to transfer in was accompanied by a sense of loss for a planned birth experience and a sense of trepidation and vulnerability over what to expect next. Given these circumstances, Jo's reception on delivery suite did nothing to alleviate any of her concerns and, in fact, reinforced her fears.

Reflecting on Jo's birth experience, outlined in Vignette 2, I would suggest that the hostility we experienced when we transferred in

Arrival on labour ward was as difficult as the strained nature of the transfer phone call had intimated. Faces peered at us over the midwives' desk as we came in – no real welcome, just staring. Once we were in a delivery room we were joined by two midwives, one friendly, one openly hostile. Unfortunately for Jo and Tony, the friendly midwife went away and we were left with the hostile one. It was hard to tell whether the disapproval was aimed at Jo, Tony, me or all of us.

While we waited for a doctor, a range of sniping comments was directed at the three of us. The atmosphere in the room was charged with tension, until Jo had a forceps delivery and there was a change of staff when she was subsequently taken down to the postnatal ward.

had more to do with the underlying clash of systems and philosophies of care than with any particular individual involved in the situation. Davis Floyd and Sargent (1997) would contextualise this within the technocratic framework of modern childbirth. For independent midwives, it represents the difficulty of mediating between relational midwifery and institutional midwifery in an environment where you are treated as an outsider and you move from being midwife to birth supporter. Leap (2000) writes that, when women need to give birth with the support of obstetric technology, our active recognition of their courage and endurance has potentially empowering conse-quences for the early transition into motherhood. Kirkham (2000) identified that organisational and medical care aims should incorpo-rate the aims of individual women. However, she observes that there is invariably a tension between the aims of the individual and the generalised provision of care. For the independent midwife working on the outside of a system, yet still connected to it by the needs of her clients, this tension is often very apparent. Jo, Tony and I perceived the experience of labour ward as alienating and disem-powering. Fortunately for Jo and Tony, the negative perceptions of the hospital system were counterbalanced by their positive experiences with the midwives on the postnatal ward.

For independent practice to work well for both midwives and women, it is essential to be able to work with other health professionals in responding to the changing needs of women during their childbearing experiences.

When we arrived, the staff were reassuring and friendly. The midwife I handed over to went through the notes and listened to what Bronwyn and Iain had to say, making a point of finding out what they had written in their birth plan. When the consultant came in to see Bronwyn, she was very friendly and interested, again asking them about their plans for the labour. The atmosphere in the room was positive, calm and caring. Ewan was delivered by forceps, and the consultant made sure that Iain was still able to cut the cord and that Bronwyn had Ewan straightaway for a first breastfeed.

Bronwyn did not have the birth she planned, but she later commented that she felt satisfied with the decisions that were made and with the care she received. She had a known midwife with her all the time, and when she transferred into hospital she felt involved in all the decision-making, supported by everyone involved. As Bronwyn's midwife, I felt that there was a partnership between the couple, the hospital staff and me. There were no underlying care conflicts or ideology clashes, but rather a cooperative approach to ensure the best outcome.

Conclusion

Becoming an independent midwife made me remember why I wanted to be a midwife in the first place. I wanted a job that would let me use my heart and mind, rather than one where I had to sell my soul just to survive. The thought of independent practice being made illegal because of the lack of political will to address insurance issues will leave women with fewer choices and, for me and many others, it will remove the fire from the heart of midwifery.

Commentary

Through her vignettes and reflection on them, Nessa provides a very clear picture of what being an independent midwife is about. Out of her account of her wealth of experience emerge the joys and the challenges of independent practice. These include her, perhaps inadvertent, picture of support in and for midwifery.

Particularly important is Nessa's picture of the mutual support that independent midwives provide for each other. Implicit in her account of the labour ward experience, though, is the less than fulsome support that independent midwives receive from some of their co-professionals working in the NHS.

Nessa refers only briefly to the appalling withdrawal of support for independent midwives by the midwifery professional organisation in 1994, which is also alluded to by Allison in her biography.

I do not overstate the case when I assert that the support of independent midwives is absolutely crucial, not only to these midwives as individual practitioners, but also to midwifery as a profession. I would argue that support is needed for the *concept* of independent practice, because it represents the autonomy and highest standards of practice to which all midwives should aspire. Rather than the 'witch hunt' to which Nessa refers, independent midwives should be embraced, encouraged and celebrated.

Independent midwives are under threat, due to what Nessa terms 'concerns about insurance'; such a threat should give rise to serious foreboding about the future of midwifery as a profession.

References

Davis-Floyd, R. and Sargent, C.F. (eds) (1997) *Childbirth and Authoritative Knowledge: Cross Cultural Perspectives*, Berkeley, CA: University of California Press.

Hobbs, L. (1997) *The Independent Midwife: A guide to independent midwifery practice*, 2nd edition, Hale: Books for Midwives.

Independent Midwives UK (IM-UK) (2008) www.independentmidwives.org.uk/ (accessed 4 May 2009).

Kaufmann, T. (2004) 'Introducing feminism', in Stewart, M. (ed.) *Pregnancy, Birth and Maternity Care: Feminist perspectives*, Edinburgh: Books for Midwives, pp. 1–10.

Kirkham, M. (ed.) (2000) *The Midwife–Mother Relationship*, Basingstoke: Macmillan.

Lawrence Beech, B.A. and Phipps, B. (2008) 'Normal birth: women's stories', in Downe, S. (ed.) *Normal Birth: Evidence and debate*, 2nd edition, Edinburgh: Churchill Livingstone, pp. 67–79.

Leap, N. (2000) 'The less we do the more we give', in Kirkham, M. (ed.) *The Midwife–Mother Relationship*, Basingstoke: Macmillan, pp. 1–18.

Pilley Edwards, N. (2000) 'Women planning homebirths: their own views on their relationships with midwives', in Kirkham, M. (ed.) *The Midwife–Mother Relationship*, Basingstoke: Macmillan, pp. 55–91.

van der Hulst, L.A.M. (1999) 'Dutch midwives: relational care and birth location', *Health and Social Care in the Community* 7: 242–7.

Wagner, M. (2004) 'A global witch hunt', *Midwifery Matters* 100, Spring: 36.

Chapter 13

A male midwife's perspective

Denis Walsh

Sally was a friend I had met through my local church. She had suffered from ME (myalgic encephalomyelitis) for over a decade, during which time she was unemployed, though she was highly qualified. I lost touch with her when I moved to another part of the city, but had heard that she had married in her late thirties. Then, out of the blue, I got a phone call from her to say that she was pregnant and asking if I would be her midwife. I was working as a Team Leader midwife and had begun to develop a small personal caseload. I enthusiastically agreed. Sally wanted a home water birth, which I was very happy to support her with, although she was 39 and still suffered with ME, whose main symptoms were excessive fatigue and lethargy. The obstetrician did not raise any objections, although I knew she was pessimistic that the labour would be straightforward. I did all the antenatal care at Sally's home and observed over the course of the pregnancy a remission in her ME symptoms. She was genuinely excited about the baby and birth and went into labour on a bright, sunny morning in May.

After a reasonably quick first stage and a three-hour second stage, Sally gave birth to a robust baby boy in the pool. It was a magic moment. The French doors to the garden were open, the sun was streaming through and we could hear children playing in the adjacent park during the labour. She did not lack energy during the labour, pushed with great gusto and had an uneventful postnatal period. She was a confident, instinctive mother. I remember driving home after the birth, feeling proud and elated that I had facilitated a birth that I am sure would have been interventionist in a maternity hospital. In the 1990s, an elderly primigravida with a history of a debilitating condition would not have been seen as a good candidate for a home birth. For me, it was the realisation of an ideal regarding what being a midwife was all about: personalised, supportive, empathic care for a woman according to her needs and her choices. I had not witnessed a medical event, but one of nature's marvels – human childbirth in the perfect setting. She had done it and I was the privileged bystander. To this day, I understand her experience as a healing one. The woman she was at the beginning of pregnancy was not the confident mother she became. She had gone on a transformatory journey and it was beautiful to witness.

Reflection

Although I had been a midwife for about five years before having this experience, I don't think I had really understood what being a midwife was truly about until then. I had been drawn to midwifery because of the autonomy of the role and the fact that its focus was not illness. In my early years of practice, exclusively in a large maternity hospital, I found that autonomy hard to realise. In addition, although everyone talked about normal birth, most of what I saw and experienced was not normal. I was living with considerable dissonance and, during those years, my practice was mostly about resistance to the biomedical model and the steady accumulation of physiological birth skills within the relative privacy of the birth room. That prepared me for the opportunity outlined above.

However, the experience of Sally's birth reordered my priorities, for the experience was not about my autonomy, but Sally's, and not about my skills, but hers. It was the first time I really understood what 'being with woman' was all about and its impact was profound. Since that time, I have pursued a teaching and research career that gave me the opportunity to research this area in the context of birth centres and to challenge midwives to reflect critically on their intrapartum practice through workshops and seminars.

Last year, I discovered 'ontology', the wonderfully rich philosophical tradition that addresses what it means 'to be', to exist – what constitutes reality. This tradition sits alongside the other great philosophical theory, epistemology, which asks the question: how do we know and what constitutes knowledge? To a researcher, epistemology is a very important theory, because it gets to the root of the kind of research and knowledge you are endeavouring to uncover or establish. What was fascinating to me was being confronted with this more fundamental question of what does it mean to be a midwife – what is its purpose and intent? The answer to this should surely inform the kind of knowledge that would be most relevant to one's ontology of midwifery. The search for an ontology of midwifery takes you back to the original derivation of the word 'midwife', which is, of course, 'with woman'. I can now call this an ontological 'presence'. That was what I experienced at Sally's birth over 15 years ago now. A search of the literature, especially around labour care, reveals a similar dynamic. Researchers speak of 'being with' not 'doing to' (Fahy 1998), 'the less we do, the more we give' (Leap 2000), 'doing nothing well' (Kennedy 2000) and 'drinking tea intelligently' (Anderson 2000).

The kind of knowledge that serves this orientation is more intuitive, though not necessarily less scientific. Knowledge from the sciences helps midwives understand physiology and the appropriate use of birth interventions. Knowledge generated by randomised controlled trials of place of birth (home, birth centres) and style of care (continuity, continuous support) assists in optimising the conditions for normal birth. Intuition is broad enough to encompass these knowledge sources, but crucially also implies a holistic appreciation of context and a profound connection with women (Fry 2007).

Thus, my experience with Sally vindicated my original 'call' to become a midwife, although it set a chain of events in motion that changed forever how I understand that call now.

My story of being a male midwife has had other challenging dimensions . . .

Aspects of lived experience of being a male midwife

During my training, I rationalised that what I 'brought to the table' as a male midwife was no different from what the childless female midwife brought: their humanity, compassion, empathy and interpersonal skills. It was not until I started to read feminist critiques of childbirth and feminist literature more widely that I realised this was a rather naive position. Of course, gender mediates care encounters and, no matter how sensitive one is to women's responses, just being male can imbue scenarios with power differentials that disadvantage women. This awareness is so important that I now believe that knowledge of feminist critiques of childbirth is not an optional extra for a male midwife. Along with Schacht and Ewing (1997), I believe it forms one of four key challenges if a male midwife is to practise with integrity. The other challenges are to reflexively consider what he, as an individual, and men as a group do to oppress women; to consider ways to reject traditional notions of masculinity that are oppressive to others and to consider feminist values and ethics as a referent for personal practice. Finally, Schacht and Ewing urge male practitioners to consider ways to place women's needs as equal or greater than their own . I have found these considerations helpful in approaching and understanding what it means for me to be a midwife, to care for women and to work with female midwifery colleagues.

Pragmatically, I apply this in practice by having sensitive antennae to women's discomfort zones when I turn up as their carer. Often they may state their preference for a female attendant, but even if I can only detect non-verbal behaviours that display this discomfort, I will offer to be replaced with a female colleague. Male midwife colleagues take an even more proactive position by requesting female midwives to inform women in advance that they have a male colleague on the team and that it is acceptable to decline his care. I did not take this route, because I thought that it might be interpreted by women that I was also uncomfortable. As I was the first male midwife to train and work locally, I wanted to communicate that I was at ease with the intimacy of the midwife–woman relationship. Because of this desire, I prioritise rapport building with women when I first meet them. I approach the task of forming interpersonal relationships by having an informal, easygoing style.

Personally, I see the relationship as akin to what Page (1995) called 'a professional friendship', mutually disclosing, as friends would, when this seems appropriate. I am not uncomfortable with the expression of emotions that regularly occurs in birth, nor with the use of touch to support or empathise with women. Touch, though, has to be measured and considered. I would not, for example, hold a woman in an embrace beyond a brief hug, although I know female midwives who do this with great effect, depending on the situation. As a rule of thumb, I don't undertake vaginal examinations unless the woman has a companion with her and I use a non-touch technique when advising on positioning for breastfeeding. Trust and rapport are very important for care encounters in pregnancy and childbirth and, for this reason, I prefer models of care that give space for their development. With those in place, the appropriate backdrop for intimate examinations exists. For these reasons, chaperoning by another member of staff is not required in my view.

One aspect I am regularly asked about in relation to caring for women in labour is how their male partners react. Rarely, in my experience, do men object to me being the midwife. When they do, it usually because of cultural or religious prohibitions or, less commonly, because they dislike their partners being cared for by a man. As when women show some disquiet, when this occurs with men, I immediately withdraw. Once I had built a good rapport with a woman over several hours of labour (she had her mother with her) until her partner turned up near the end of the labour. When I was relieved for a break, he told the midwife that he did not want me attending his partner, so I withdrew. After the baby was born, I went in to to see her (the partner had left by then) and she was crying. She said she was mortified at his earlier actions and thought it would have really upset me. I reassured her that was not the case, but clearly he was unable to cope with having a male attendant.

Usually, I have a very good relationship with a male birth companion and take the time to get to know him by seeking common areas to converse on. Although this probably puts him at ease, it is not always helpful for the birth room atmosphere. Conversation and attention diverted to others in the birth room can be distracting for the woman and could compromise my own observation and connection with her. Generally, I take those opportunities in early labour but not as labour progresses. The other interesting dimension in relation to male partners occurs in couple childbirth preparation classes. Over the years, together with female colleagues, we have split the classes on gender lines at particular junctures and I have facilitated the men talking about their experiences of the antenatal period. Gradually, they start to share worries and concerns, often with respect to relationship tensions. These sessions have been well evaluated by men and expose unmet needs in this group, which latterly the Fatherhood Institute (2008) has taken forward.

As good as a female midwife?

What has troubled me more over the years is whether I can support women in labour as well as my female colleagues. A male midwife friend eventually left the profession and one of the aspects he particularly struggled with was how patronising he felt when verbally encouraging women through the intensity of labour. Knowing he could never share this experience made him feel his words were patronising and paternalistic. Of course, one could argue that childless female midwives may feel the same, but at least they share the same reproductive biology. As I read about intuition and heard stories of highly intuitive midwives, I was concerned that there was some female reservoir of wisdom and insight that I could never tap into as a man.

Around the same time, feminist scholarship was beginning to challenge gender essentialism (Annandale and Clark 1996), as postmodern ideas were explored. Postmodern perspectives challenge taken-for-granted assumptions behind discourses such as the biomedical model, capitalism, democracy, etc. In the same way, they challenge the idea that men and women think and act differently (Gray 1992), arguing that differences are socially constructed and serve to reinforce stereotypes and roles. This opened up the possibility that intuitive skills could be modelled or accrued through mentoring and observation and were not fixed as female-only characteristics.

It could be argued that many of what might be considered the characteristics of good care – listening skills, empathy, kindness, sensitivity to individual needs, up-to-date knowledge, clinical skills – are generic across genders. There is an additional and important dimension that links to intuitive care, but is not the same as that which has been popularised in contemporary management and self-help literature – emotional intelligence (Goleman 1996). My own research into the work of staff in birth centres suggests that birth attendants there utilise emotional intelligence in the care of women to great effect. I hypothesised this as 'matrescent' (becoming mother) care, which is a subtle blend of comforting, encouraging, enabling and leaving alone (Walsh 2006). Hunter (2005) and Dahlen (2008) also write about the importance of emotional work by midwives. This kind of sensitivity is related to having a high degree of self-awareness, competence and confidence in relationships and being comfortable with the intimacy and embodied aspects of childbirth. All of these are unlikely to be the preserve of women only.

Apart from positive feedback from women about the effectiveness of my care, these ideas have helped sustain me in clinical practice.

Conflict and gender

What I did not anticipate in my career as a midwife was conflict with male obstetricians that would significantly influence my decision to leave full-time practice. Again, feminist critique has illuminated gender games in the workplace, in particular the doctor–nurse game in health: the female nurse has a great idea to improve care, but to implement it she has to sell it to the male doctor so that he takes ownership of it (Sweet and Norman 1995). Part of her selling technique may involve flirtatious behaviours and 'friendly banter'. That game has strong resonances with what I have observed in maternity units, but it has obvious limitations when the midwife is male. I was told an amended version by a male health service manager. He recommended building a 'blokey rapport' with male consultants (conversations around sport, cars, drinking exploits), so that you are on first-name terms. The next step is to present new ideas as solutions to existing problems, so that doctors' lives will be easier. He can then get on with his job of expert clinician without management interference.

These strategies have more than a touch of compromising one's integrity and buying into unhelpful power relationships and hierarchies that will remain unchallenged. At the extreme end of these manipulative behaviours and compliance with the status quo may be bullying and intimidation, which is allowed to continue. For all these reasons, I never took this path and, as a consequence, encountered conflict regularly with some obstetricians. I also experienced professional bullying, which was instrumental in my decision to leave clinical practice, although not before an exit interview during which I spoke with candour. The professor apologised for his actions.

Territorial disputes

Complicating gender politics in maternity care are historical professional struggles between obstetrics and midwifery. These transcend gender and are, therefore, played out between female midwives and obstetricians and male midwives and male obstetricians, as described above. My own view is that a lot of these conflicts are accentuated by the context of institutional care in large busy hospitals. Where space is made for building trust and mutual understanding, a true partnership in care can emerge and a positive interdisciplinary environment can flourish. Along with Downe *et al.* (2007), I don't believe that pigeon-holing obstetricians or midwives as anti- or pro-normal birth is helpful or even accurate, and the most creative and best maternity services exist where the common ground is shared.

Having said that, the potent effect of professional groups' socialisation often results in midwives who lack autonomy and the assertiveness skills to address this (Ball *et al.* 2003). Many midwives hear themselves being referred to as 'my midwives', or experts in meeting psychosocial needs, but marginalised from real clinical autonomy in their dealings with obstetricians. There are several strategies that I think are helpful in remedying this. One is the mandatory teaching of assertiveness skills, using role play and reflection, for all student midwives. A second is investing in continuity models of working, based in primary care. The experience of autonomy is facilitated by the independence that can be realised from a primary care base. Hand in hand with autonomy goes accountability and midwives need nurturing into accepting these twin professional responsibilities. It is only from a secure sense of one's own skill base and confidence in one's role that relationships of equality with other professional groups can be entered into. I have observed great examples of positive interprofessional working between midwives and obstetricians in recent years and this needs modelling and replicating more widely.

One strategic feature that would assist midwifery's self-confidence is obtaining representation in the more strategic local NHS Trust posts, such as Clinical Director or Chief Executive. At the moment, there are two Clinical Directors in England who are midwives and no Chief Executives. Very senior posts in the NHS are gendered, reflecting the under-representation of women in senior management posts more broadly in society (Moore and Buttner 1997). It was very encouraging to read Byrom and Downe's (2008) paper on transformational leadership in midwifery. These are exactly the kinds of posts, individuals and styles of leadership that can help the profession out of its historical inferiority to medicine.

Academic life as a male midwife

Although my exposure to feminist literature and scholarship has occurred since I have worked in universities, I can honestly say that, in the main, other (female) midwifery academics have been very welcoming and inclusive. Even those who had previously published their reservations about the entry of men into the profession have been supportive and encouraging. About eight years ago, in the midst of doubts about my continued contribution to midwifery as a man, two experiences convinced me that I could make a worthwhile contribution. One was the reception and feedback I received from the launch of an evidence course in normal labour and birth, which has subsequently been attended by over 3,000 midwives in many countries. The second was an invitation to contribute a chapter to an edited book about feminist perspectives on pregnancy and childbirth (Stewart 2003). That another midwife could think I could have some input into such a book was amazing. Since then, I have felt more at ease with writing and speaking about the ongoing important contribution feminist scholarship is making to midwifery and childbirth issues.

Being a male researcher interviewing exclusively female research participants has raised a number of issues for me. There was a time when I thought that my gender would prohibit me from doing childbirth research. If Oakley, a pioneering feminist, struggled with the idea of researching women's experience, as she debates in the thought-provoking chapter 'Interviewing women: a contradiction in terms' (Oakley 1981), then how could a man?

One of the issues was the whole notion of being a researcher first and a person second in relation to data collection and interactions with people in the field. Others with feminist sensitivities have construed this dilemma as 'faking friendship' (Duncombe and Jessop 2002) and this phrase captures the ambivalence it creates for the researcher. In the textbooks, one of the dangers of ethnographic field-work includes the possibility of 'going native', where identification with the observed group reaches a point where the outsider perspective is lost (Donovan 2005). I found myself dropping the researcher persona, and relating quite spontaneously and naturally. It occurred several months into fieldwork and reflected the fact that I was forming relationships with the staff and that an easy familiarity was evolving. Instead of me listening and observing, I was starting to tell stories and generally reveal more of myself to them.

The challenge in these situations is to achieve congruence between one's authenticity and genuineness and the need to remain a researcher first. Achieving a sense of congruence is not just for one's own integrity, but also out of respect for those being contacted in the field. Feminist writers particularly put a high value on this, with their central concern being to diminish power differentials between the researcher and the research participant.

Conclusion

It is interesting to speculate about the popularity of midwifery as a career option for men. I suspect that the numbers of men entering the profession have not changed that much since Lewis's (1991) original survey of nearly 20 years ago. It may be because the male midwife has high visibility within the service and this results in a level of scrutiny that many men would not welcome. Or because the nature of the work is simply unappealing, although this begs the question as to why obstetrics and gynaecology remain relatively popular with male doctors.

High visibility can be an advantage if the male midwife is popular with staff and clients but, equally, perceived shortcomings precede you wherever you go. Early on in my training I was once greeted with, 'I heard you were quite normal'!

I have no regret about my decision to become a midwife. It has provided some of the most memorable experiences of my life and, through it, I have met many remarkable people, both fellow midwives and mothers. Of course, I have concerns about the medicalisation of childbirth, the semi-autonomous, and not often enough fully autonomous, nature of our role and the effects of an institutional model on women. However, the privilege of witnessing and attending physiological birth, with all its challenge, courage and emotion, sustains me. Oh, and of course the discovery of ontological presence as a midwife's *raison d'être*.

Commentary

I feel rather wary of the term 'male midwife', but Denis chose the title of his chapter and I use it for that reason. My concern with this term relates to my fear of labelling the midwife simply on the basis of gender. I would prefer to consider him as 'a midwife who is a man'. In my view, this would recognise that he has a wide range of other characteristics, in addition to his gender. The term 'male midwife' may have the effect of excluding or even denying this midwife's compassion, insight and integrity – to name but a few additional qualities.

In the same way, I am wary of labelling others, particularly those for whom the midwife provides care. For example, if a woman has diabetes, she is likely to be referred to as a 'diabetic mother'. If you take the time to tap this phrase into your favourite search engine, you'll find how frequently and by what authoritative sources this term is used. What does such a term say about the way that we view this woman? Does it mean that all we see when we meet her is the diabetes-related problems? Is it possible to see her enthusiasm to assume some control over her experience of birth? Or her wish to breastfeed her baby immediately after birth?

Such labelling features in any number of ways in midwifery care and in maternity. A particularly recalcitrant example that persists, despite the efforts of a range of midwifery writers, is the term 'patient' being used to describe the childbearing woman (Thomson 1999). What does this word say about the midwife's view of the woman whom he or she attends? It may say that the midwife is using a jargon term, which means nothing more than that the woman is being given care in hospital. Or, like Parsons (1951), it may say that the midwife regards childbearing as a health problem, or even an illness, requiring a range of interventions. The term 'patient' carries with it a range of rights and obligations that are inherent in the 'sick role'. These feature a submissiveness that has no place in the behaviour of the childbearing woman.

Similarly, I would argue that the term 'male midwife' carries the danger of reducing the humanity of the person providing care. This issue re-emerges in the closing paragraphs of Denis's chapter, when he recounts the greeting, 'I heard you were quite normal'!

What was this person actually saying? This greeting may have been referring to the fact that he has only one head. I am inclined to question, though, whether it may mean something altogether more disturbing. While our nursing cousins have addressed their widespread stereotypes of male nurses as gay (Evans 2002; Harding 2007), this is something that UK midwives seem to be reluctant to discuss, although students are beginning to open up the topic (StudentMidwife.Net 2008). Keeping discussion of gender orientation so firmly under wraps cannot be a healthy situation for midwifery or a helpful approach to our colleagues who are gay.

References

Anderson, T. (2000) 'Feeling safe enough to let go: the relationship between the woman and her midwife in the second stage of labour', in Kirkham, M. (ed.) *The Midwife–Woman Relationship*, London: Routledge, pp. 92–118.

Annandale, E. and Clark, J. (1996) What is gender? Feminist theory and the sociology of human reproduction, *Sociology of Health and Illness* 18: 17–44.

Ball, L., Curtis, P. and Kirkham, M. (2003) *Why Do Midwives Leave?*, London: Royal College of Midwives.

Byrom, S. and Downe, S. (2008) ' "She sort of shines": midwives' accounts of "good" midwifery and "good" leadership', *Midwifery*, June.

Dahlen, H. (2008) 'The novice birthing: theorising first-time mothers' experiences of birth at home and in hospital in Australia', *Midwifery*, June.

Donovan, P. (2005) 'Ethnography', in Cluett, E. and Bluff, R. (eds) *Principles and Practice of Research in Midwifery*, London: Baillière Tindall, pp. 171–185.

Downe, S., Mckeown, M. and Johnston, E. (2007) 'The UCLan community engagement and service user support (Comensus) project: valuing authenticity, making space for emergence', *Health Expectations* 10(4): 392–406.

Duncombe, J. and Jessop, J. (2002) ' "Doing rapport" and the ethics of "faking friendship" ', in Mauthner, M., Birch, M., Jessop, J. and Miller, T. (eds) *Ethics in Qualitative Research*, London: Sage, pp. 107–22.

Evans, J.A. (2002) 'Cautious caregivers: gender stereotypes and the sexualization of men nurses' touch', *Journal of Advanced Nursing* 40(4): 441–8.

Fahy, K. (1998) 'Being a midwife or doing midwifery', *Australian Midwives College Journal* 11(2): 11–16.

Fatherhood Institute (2008) *The Dad Deficit: The missing piece of the maternity jigsaw*, London: DHA Communications.

Fry, J. (2007) 'Are there other ways of knowing? An explanation of intuition as a source of authoritative knowledge in childbirth', *MIDIRS Midwifery Digest* 17(3): 325–8.

Goleman, D. (1996) *Emotional Intelligence*, London: Bloomsbury.

Gray, J. (1992) *Men are from Mars, Women are from Venus*, London: Bloomsbury.

Harding, T. (2007) 'The construction of men who are nurses as gay', *Journal of Advanced Nursing* 60(6): 636–44.

Hunter, B. (2005) 'Emotion work and boundary maintenance in hospital-based midwifery, *Midwifery* 21(3): 253–66.

Kennedy, H. (2000) 'A model of exemplary midwifery practice: results of a Delphi study, including commentary by Ernst K', *Journal of Midwifery & Women's Health* 45(1): 4–19.

Leap, N. (2000) 'The less we do, the more we give', in Kirkham, M. (ed.) *The Midwife–Mother Relationship*, London: Macmillan, pp. 1–18.

Lewis, P. (1991) 'Men in midwifery: their experiences as students and practitioners', in Robinson, S. and Thomson, A. (eds) *Midwives, Research and Childbirth, Vol. 2*, London: Chapman and Hall.

Moore, D. and Buttner, E. (1997) *Moving Beyond the Glass Ceiling*, London: Sage.

Oakley, A. (1981) 'Interviewing women: a contradiction in terms', in Roberts, H. (ed.) *Doing Feminist Research*, London: Routledge, pp.123–41.

Page, L. (1995) 'Putting principles into practice', in Page, L. (ed.) *Effective Group Practice in Midwifery: Working with women*, Oxford: Blackwell Science, pp. 12–17.

Parsons, T. (1951) 'Illness and the role of the physician: a sociological perspective', *American Journal of Orthopsychiatry* 21: 452–60.

Schacht, S. and Ewing, S. (1997) 'The many paths of feminism: can men travel any of them?' *Journal of Gender Studies* 6(2): 159–76.

StudentMidwife.Net (2008) *Lesbian Midwives/Student Midwives*. Available online at www.studentmidwife.net/student-midwife-discussion/1052-lesbian-midwives-student-midwives.html#post5114 (accessed 7 January 2009).

Sweet, S. and Norman, I. (1995) 'The nurse–doctor relationship: a selective literature review', *Journal of Advanced Nursing* 22: 165–70.

Stewart, M. (2003) *Pregnancy, Birth and Maternity Care: Feminist perspectives*, London: Books for Midwives.

Thomson, A. (1999) 'The importance of the words we used', *Midwifery* 15(2): 65.

Walsh, D. (2006) '"Nesting" and "matrescence": distinctive features of a free-standing birth centre', *Midwifery* 22(3): 228–39.

Chapter 14

The midwife who is not a mother

Rosemary Mander

Introduction

In this chapter, I reflect on what it is like to be a midwife who is not a mother. To do this, I draw mainly on my own experience of being a midwife who is childfree, that is, voluntarily childless. It is possible that some of the ideas I present here may also apply to the midwife who is childless; this means that, for some reason outside her control, she doesn't have children. This latter group would include the midwife who is involuntarily infertile, as well as the midwife whose child(ren) have been miscarried or who have died.

In order to contemplate the experience of the midwife who is not a mother, I start with a report of the first part of a conversation with a new mother. I have called her Catriona, although that is not her real name. This report is followed immediately by an account of the ensuing encounter with my midwifery colleagues. Before reflecting on this conversation, I describe the demographic changes that provide the context for this discussion. I next reflect on what was happening in my conversation with Catriona and the subsequent encounter with my colleagues. My reflection is followed by the second part of the first vignette, which comprises an account of the latter part of my conversation with Catriona. In this, I seek to address some of the issues raised in my reflection. In order to draw to a conclusion my view of the experience of the midwife who is not a mother, the concluding vignette comprises a quite different scenario. This final part provides an account of an interaction between a childbearing woman, for whom I was providing care, and another health professional who was a mother.

Working in the ward on a day when it was functioning at something less than its usual frantic pace, I was able to take a little time to get to know Catriona and her baby, Seona. While I had been doing her 'obs', Catriona had been looking at my left hand and noticed that I was wearing a wedding ring.

After talking about her plans for going home later in the day and how she should best prepare herself and her family, she asked me the not totally unexpected question: 'How many children do you have?' I replied with my stock answer: ''Fraid I don't have any. I've never quite got around to it. We've been too busy doing other things.'

Catriona and I looked at each other.

She was clearly wondering about whether she should have asked the question in the first place. At the same time, I found myself worrying about whether I'd deflected her enquiry in a sufficiently laid-back manner.

(My conversation with Catriona continued and the remainder is recounted below in the vignette on pages 187–8.)

A short while later, in the coffee room, I mentioned to the other midwives that the question was asked and I mused aloud about what it means and whether I could have dealt with it in a better way. My colleagues were quite accustomed to my musings. Such ramblings were usually dealt with by means of a quite lighthearted dismissal. On this occasion, though, I soon realised that something was different. I seemed to have touched a raw nerve and I found that my musings were greeted with an embarrassed silence. Looking around at the others, I quickly became aware that I was the only midwife sitting at the table who was not actually a mother. My colleagues, though, were unwilling to articulate to me what they were all thinking. This was their belief that, to be a 'proper midwife', it is necessary to have completed certain personal experiences. This is what, in the days of the two-part midwifery training, used to be called 'Part Three'; which means to have given birth to a child and to have become a mother.

Reflection

The first part of this brief vignette shows that the midwife having had personal childbearing experience matters, both to the child-bearing woman and to the midwife caring for her. In order to help with my reflection on this vignette, it may be useful to distinguish the views of the midwife or midwives from those of the woman. I recognise that such a distinction may be quite artificial. I hope, though, that it will help me to tease apart what is happening when this question is, first, asked by the woman; second, answered by the childfree midwife; and, third, reacted to by the midwives who are mothers.

The demographic context

There have long been assumptions about women's destinies being intertwined with their childbearing capability. These assumptions have given rise to concepts such as 'maternal instinct', as well as occasional pronatalist policies. In the latter part of the twentieth century, the socio-demographic picture began to change. The much-publicised 'baby boom' of the 1960s meant that women born in the 1930s would complete their families with an average of 2.46 children (Social Trends 2004). Since then, completed family size has declined in the UK to an average of about 1.74 children for women born in the mid-1980s. This picture is variably reflected throughout Europe, being most noticeable in Germany.

This image of declining family size is partly attributable to an increasing proportion of women without children. For women born in 1945, the number of women without children was as low as 9 per cent. This figure has risen to almost 20 per cent for women currently completing their reproductive lives. There are signs, however, that total fertility rates have bottomed out and that fertility is beginning to increase (Social Trends 2008). Such published material, though, is not yet clear about whether there is any association with women remaining childless or childfree. As Park (2002) recognises, interpreting these data is far from straightforward, due to the problems of obtaining accurate data on the reasons why people do not have children. There is difficulty differentiating between the celibate, those who are physically unable to have children, those who are delaying childbearing and those who are childless by choice.

The childbearing woman's question

It is necessary to dismiss, first of all, the possibility that the woman asking about the midwife's personal childbearing experience is just making small talk. The new mother has far too much on her mind to be concerned with such fripperies. If she manages to bring herself to ask a question, it is because she has a purpose, an agenda or some issue that she really needs to get sorted out.

Possible reasons for the question may relate to the likelihood that Catriona was seeking to find a basis for our working relationship. This basis may have involved her search for shared values or, at least, common ground on which we could both build some degree of understanding, empathy or even rapport. Some commonality or similar background would help in establishing that we were both at least speaking the same language. Following on from this, we would be able to engage in conversation at a level that is something other than patently superficial.

Another, perhaps associated, reason for the question relates to the possibility of Catriona testing out my credentials. This would be more than the obvious fact of my being qualified as a midwife. It was this fact that underpinned my greeting when I introduced myself to her. Through her question, she could have been trying to find out the depth or extent to which I was qualified, if I was to provide effective care for her and Seona. As is so often the case, Catriona was falling into the trap of equating experience with expertise. She was asking whether I was really sufficiently knowledgeable to be trusted, or were my qualifications nothing more than bits of paper. It may be that neither paper qualifications nor occupational experience nor personal childbearing experience are sufficient by themselves to facilitate effective midwifery practice. Each of these forms of experience is only able to enhance the standard of the midwife's practice if she allows herself to learn from it. It is the learning from experience and the application of that learning to practice that really leads to genuine midwifery expertise.

Building on from this deeper level of knowledge, Catriona could have been searching for a specific form of care to meet her needs as a new mother. She may have been seeking a common experience, which would ensure that I was able to offer her empathy at a time when shared understandings really mattered to her. This shared experience or orientation may equate with the 'motherliness' to which Thomas refers as protecting the new mother from the 'unfamiliar and sometimes unfriendly world' (1994: 3). Walsh has developed this concept of the motherly role of the midwife and he summarises it by using the word 'matrescence'. He describes the role in terms of being 'protective, nurturing' (2007: 103), which carries the promise of security and is calm and reassuring, rather like a warm, friendly hug.

A further possible reason for the question is highly relevant in the UK in the twenty-first century, when mobile and nuclear families are so prevalent. This is the likelihood that Catriona might actually have been looking for a role model on which to base her perception of herself as a mother. Catriona was living a considerable distance away from her own mother and sisters, and she had become somewhat isolated during her period of employment. As a result, her contact with other childbearing women was seriously limited. Thus, identifying somebody who had been through this experience and had come out the other side may have provided her with evidence that she, too, was capable of a similar achievement.

In this way, Catriona is likely to have been asking her seriously meaningful question for one or more of a whole range of reasons.

The childfree midwife's answer

What was I doing in giving my answer to Catriona's all-too-familiar question? Was I really just mouthing my usual stock reply? Was my purpose merely to deflect her curiosity away from my personal, domestic circumstances and back on to matters that were my reason for being with her, that is, to provide care for Catriona and Seona?

As the first part of the vignette shows, I was not able just to reply 'None' and move on to talk about other things. I found that it was necessary for me to embellish, explain and perhaps rationalise my position, which Catriona may have thought surprising, or even disconcerting. The very fact that I had to defend my childfree status speaks volumes about the sensitivity of this subject for midwives. This was one of the findings of Bewley's insightful research project, which looked at midwives who do not have children. She reports her finding that midwives 'needed to justify their response' (2000a:137). This justification, though, sometimes resorted to humour as a coping strategy, such as making references to wanting to sleep at night, or to pets as child-substitutes.

As well as trying to redirect our conversation away from my personal circumstances, I was also seeking to show Catriona that the well-known negative stereotypes of childfree women are in no way applicable to me. It was only about 50 years ago that being childfree started to become a realistic option; since then, there have been any number of research projects to examine the position of childfree people. These studies have clearly and consistently demonstrated the 'bad press' with which childfree women and couples are faced (Mander 1996; Gillespie 2003; Koropeckyj-Cox et al. 2007). The rationale underpinning such persistently negative perceptions, which probably constitute stereotypes, is not entirely clear. In her perceptive paper, Gillespie (2003) suggests that such negative attributes may be being applied to people who choose to not accept, or possibly even reject, the child-centred values that are prevalent in our society. She goes on to advance the argument that being childfree is widely regarded as 'deviant, unhealthy and unfeminine and . . . transgresses traditional constructions of femininity' (2003:124).

The negative characteristics perceived as attributable to the child-free state are distinguished by Park (2002) from the characteristics of the childless. It is this distinction, Park maintains, that is responsible for the effective stigmatisation of the childfree. She quotes conspiracy theorists who argue that such stigmatisation constitutes 'a mechanism to enforce parenting' (2002: 25).

Thus, in my answer to Catriona, I was trying to distance myself from such negative stereotypes, which verge on stigma. In doing this, I may also have been attempting to establish my credentials as a suitable person to provide care for her and Seona.

Thus, at the same time as I was endeavouring to demonstrate to her what I was *not*, I was also attempting to achieve a more positive outcome. This involved ensuring that I was able to maintain a high level of rapport, which would facilitate the provision of all aspects of care for this mother and baby. It could be that, had I given the wrong answer, I might have served to confirm in Catriona's mind the stereotype mentioned by Gillespie. It would also have jeopardised the working relationship that Catriona and I had begun to establish. Thus, it was crucial for me to try to answer her question in terms that would reassure her of my 'child-friendliness'. For this reason, my choice of explanation avoided too much detail, while ensuring that the effective communication that we had developed was in no way jeopardised.

A further way in which the childfree midwife may seek to ensure that such rapport is not threatened is for the midwife to actually tell lies to the woman for whom she is caring. In the report of her study, Bewley (2000a) describes this phenomenon in terms of the midwife seeking to protect her vulnerable self from inquisitive questioning. This research report mentions a midwife who 'invented' two grown-up children who were at university. The inevitable question that arises is 'Why stop at two?' A childfree colleague of mine, who is an expert in helping women to breastfeed, is in the habit of reporting having successfully breastfed all *four* of her children! My observation of fabrication by my expert colleague highlights another issue that emerged out of Bewley's study. This was the way in which it is invariably *colleagues* who dream up or invent fictitious children. It is never the person who is actually writing or answering the question. This can only lead to one conclusion. This is that the childfree midwife is likely to be less than comfortable at feeling the need to mislead the woman with whom she is trying to build a trusting relationship. Thus, the reports are invariably of others' lies.

The reactions of the other midwives

The reason for the midwives in the vignette showing such a wary reaction may have related in no small part to the long and honourable history of midwives and midwifery. Unlike our nursing cousins, whose occupational origins are found in the religious and the military, midwives originated in the neighbourly activities of women in the community. Those women who had borne children came together to provide support for other women at the time of birth. In this way, certain women became recognised as particularly knowledgeable. As a result, they were more likely to be called on for support and, possibly, more active help. Thus, midwifery's largely domestic and social origins distinguish it from other occupational groups. Through this historical background, the assumption that the midwife would have personal experience of childbearing was not only continued, but became reinforced.

The embarrassed silence I encountered in the first vignette may be associated with the midwives' feelings about their own motherhood. Unsurprisingly, the midwives, like women in general, attach great store or value to their experience as mothers and the status that the experience carries with it (Park 2002). In view of this potential for motherhood to elevate the status of the woman, there is a tendency to discount, or even dismiss, those who, for whatever reason, find themselves lacking in that experience.

This elevation of status of the mother and discounting or dismissal of the childfree is associated in midwifery with an implicit hierarchy of experience. By this I mean that no quantity or duration of occupational experience is regarded as able to compensate for the absence of personal childbearing experience. Similarly, a midwife who is a mother, even though she has accrued relatively little occupational experience, is credited with higher occupational status than her childfree colleague with many years of practice. It may be that the privileging of personal experience over other forms reflects on the position of midwifery as either an occupation or as a profession

The 'bad press' that childfree women encounter was outlined in the article cited earlier (Mander 1996). In this article, I also indicated the adverse characteristics that may be attributed to childfree women, including an insensitivity to the feelings and needs of others. That this attribution is sometimes applied to the childfree midwife (Flint 1989: 5) may not be surprising, but it is certainly disconcerting. This observation supports the contention made by Kirkham (1999) that midwives find it relatively easy to empathise with and to care for their women clients, but less easy to care for each other. The attribution of insensitivity is but one more example of the childfree midwife's 'bad press', which may lead to the assumption 'that midwives who do not have children are somehow lacking' (Bewley 2000b: 170).

After Catriona and I looked at each other questioningly for what seemed like minutes, but could not have been more than a few seconds, Catriona went on to ask, 'Well, how do you manage to be a midwife? How do you know what to do? How do you know what a mother is thinking and what she is feeling?'

How indeed? Not easily, that is quite certain.

'Well,' I replied, choosing my words carefully, 'I read a lot. I read the research and I read what mothers write about their experiences. Even more importantly, though, I listen to the women I'm working with. I listen to what they say. And I listen to what they don't say. I recognise that each woman is different – a unique individual. And that applies to her experience of becoming and being a mother, too. Because I don't have any personal experience of being a mother, I can't draw on that experience. I can't make any assumptions about the mother I'm working with. I certainly can't assume that her experience is in any way comparable with mine. I have to listen carefully to the woman and to believe what she tells me. And then I work with her on the basis of what she has and has not said.'

Conclusion

Working in the labour ward, I was caring for Lexa, a young woman who was not well supported and who had no birth companion. Having been scared, throughout her pregnancy, of the very thought of labour, Lexa decided to ask for an epidural at the earliest opportunity. Knowing that the maternity unit offered an epidural service, she planned the birth of her baby accordingly.

When Lexa was in labour, despite the best efforts of our anaesthetic colleagues, the epidural was effective only on her left side. She was suffering pain for which she had had no reason to prepare herself, either physically or emotionally.

Not surprisingly, as a result of suffering such unexpected labour pain, Lexa was bitterly disappointed and showed it very clearly in the form of anger. As a midwife, I was required to draw on my full repertoire of caring and interpersonal skills to support Lexa through this doubly negative experience.

Having exhausted the registrars' endeavours, the most senior obstetric anaesthetist was summoned to resolve the apparently intractable problem of this relatively unsupported mother's failed epidural. The consultant anaesthetist was clearly unaccustomed to such a dismal scenario. Her response verged on the defensive. It took the form of demanding of the distressed, frightened and angry young woman, 'Lexa! What the hell are you up to – making all this fuss? I've had four without an epidural and I never made all this noise.'

Commentary

In this chapter, the first vignette outlines a dialogue that is fairly commonplace between midwives and the women for whom they are caring; that of the woman enquiring as to the number of children the midwife has and the midwife apologising for not having any, followed by the subsequent embarrassment on both sides.

Rosemary continues by engaging in a frank and open discussion with her clinical midwifery colleagues about the prerequisite of motherhood for midwifery, pointing out that many did feel it necessary to have the experience of motherhood to do the job. Indeed, about 100 years ago and more, women who became midwives were women who had themselves given birth and brought up families. They were usually women who were respected in their communities for this and who could be apprenticed to their local midwife.

So what caused the change? No one thing is responsible, but it is generally attributed to the professionalisation of midwifery, when midwifery education became more prescribed and required full-time commitment. Benoit (1997) notes that this is still the situation in parts of Canada, in her article outlining three different models of midwifery education that co-exist there: apprenticeship, a three-year bachelor's programme and a master's programme for registered nurses. However, in Europe, education standards are set by the EU and each member country.

There is, of course, no easy answer to the question, but a point not addressed in the chapter is whether 'Catriona' felt that Rosemary needed to have children or to have given birth. The two do not always go together and readers need to be aware of this.

References

Benoit, C. (1997) 'Professionalizing Canadian midwifery: sociological perspectives', in Shroff, F. (ed.) *The New Midwifery: Reflections on renaissance and regulation*, Toronto: The Women's Press, pp. 93–114.

Bewley, C. (2000a) 'Feelings and experiences of midwives who do not have children about caring for childbearing women', *Midwifery* 16(2): 135–44.

Bewley, C. (2000b) 'Midwives' personal experiences and their relationships with women: midwives without children', in Kirkham, M. (ed.) *The Midwife–Mother Relationship*, London: Macmillan, Ch. 8.

Flint, C. (1989) *Sensitive Midwifery*, London: Heinemann.

Gillespie, R. (2003) 'Childfree and feminine: understanding the gender identity of voluntarily childless women', *Gender & Society* 17(1): 122–36.

Kirkham, M. (1999) 'The culture of midwifery in the National Health Service in England', *Journal of Advanced Nursing* 30(3): 732–9.

Koropeckyj-Cox, T., Romano, V. and Moras, A. (2007) 'Through the lenses of gender, race, and class: students' perceptions of childless/childfree individuals and couples', *Sex Roles* 56(7–8):415–28.

Mander, R. (1996) 'The childfree midwife: the significance of personal experience of childbearing', *Midwives* 109(1302): 186–8.

Park, K. (2002) 'Stigma management among the voluntarily childless', *Sociological Perspectives* 45:1 21–45.

Social Trends (2004) 'Completed family size'. Available online at www.statistics.gov.uk/CCI/nugget.asp?ID=762&Pos=6&ColRank=2&Rank=528 (accessed 5 November 2008).

Social Trends (2008) 'Fertility: rise in UK fertility continues'. Available online at www.statistics.gov.uk/cci/nugget.asp?id=951 (accessed 5 November 2008).

Thomas, P. (1994) 'Accountable for what? New thoughts on the midwife/mother relationship', *AIMS Journal* 6(3): 1–5.

Walsh, D. (2007) *Improving Maternity Services*, Oxford: Radcliffe Publishing.

Chapter 15

The midwife who is an author

Penny Curtis

Some years ago now, I was responsible for drafting an article for publication in an academic journal. I had been involved, with a colleague, in the evaluation of a small-scale, pilot project to establish a practice initiative. Colleagues responsible for procuring funding, planning, establishing and running the project were highly committed, both professionally and emotionally, to its success. That the project worked was, not surprisingly, important to them and they were concerned to do their best for all involved. My co-researcher and I were brought in, in the final few months of the project, when we planned and executed the realistic evaluation, reported the findings and eventually began the process of writing up elements for publication and dissemination to a broader professional and academic audience.

The article that I drafted explored the concept of empowerment and the facilitators and barriers to empowerment within the practice setting. One of the key themes that we wished to consider was the extent to which the realities of practice may lead to divergence in the nature of the involvement of members of different groups. Our evaluation suggested that the project's overarching aims and objectives became less central to the activities of some participants as new opportunities developed for them, over time.

We felt that this was an important message and that acknowledgement and discussion of the potential for such 'organic' change was of value within midwifery, suggesting as it did that what comes to *matter* about an initiative – the outcomes that people work towards – may not always be wholly predictable at the outset. Where such different outcomes become important, they have the potential to influence, positively or negatively, what happens in practice.

While some members of the project team shared our belief that this was a worthwhile issue to discuss in the academic and professional literature, we also encountered considerable opposition. We were asked to consider the implications of reporting such a finding for future funding: if we were suggesting that different parties were working to advance different objectives, would this not invalidate or at least undermine the initiative as a whole? Was there a danger that our paper might undermine the confidence of the funder in the project outcomes? We were also asked to take particular care in acknowledging the limitations of the evaluation process: concern for client confidentiality meant that the project had been set up in a way that made it difficult to access a key group of participants, or to collect a form of data that we felt would have extended the analytical potential of the evaluation.

Discussion did not resolve these issues and we were, at the time, unable to reconcile differences between interested parties. We could not find a way to write this article that did not provoke conflict with the project team: in the end, we did not submit the article for publication.

This experience raises two fundamental, though related, questions: Why should the midwife author? And are there circumstances in which midwives have a moral and/or ethical responsibility to write? I will reflect upon my own experience as I return to these questions, but first it is important to locate the midwife as an author and ask who writes and in what context?

Who is the midwife author?

The midwife author may wear a variety of hats, sometimes successively, sometimes interchangeably. Students entering the midwifery profession may have much to say about the process of socialisation as they encounter and become immersed in the world of midwifery practice. Their educational experience may cause them to reflect upon or synthesise knowledge in a new way that has the potential to inform others in the profession or spark debate. Once in practice, midwives confront, on a daily basis, clinical issues, deficits in the existing knowledge base, ethical dilemmas, ongoing research and professional development issues, which may all prompt the practising midwife to write. Managers, confronting the rapid pace of health service change and the barrage of difficulties that they encounter in attempting to deliver a quality service, may write in an effort to influence the political environment, as they witness the pressures upon those colleagues responsible for the provision of direct client care. Authorship may be fuelled by a desire to improve practitioners' working conditions and the birth experiences of childbearing women, or to demonstrate the benefits of practice initiatives that managers have introduced and supported. The health service research midwife may be obliged to publicise research methods and findings from research studies: to demonstrate benefit; to discuss lack of effect; to fulfil the requirements of funding bodies and to bolster Trust research outputs. Authorship may, therefore, be differently intentioned and any or all of these differently positioned midwives may write with an eye to career development or career change.

Perhaps uniquely, however, the midwife academic has little option but to write. Writing for publication is a core aspect of an academic role and one that many of us struggle with to a greater or lesser extent. It is from my own standpoint of authoring as part of an academic role that I continue this discussion. Though there will inevitably be differences between my own perspectives and experiences and those of colleagues writing in other roles, there will also be issues and experiences that resonate across roles.

A standpoint view – why should midwives author?

I concluded the description of one of my own authoring experiences by asking why the midwife should write. There may be 'process' reasons as well as 'outcome' reasons: by process, I refer to the 'doing' of writing – the undertaking of the task. Outcome refers to the experiences that may be associated with having accomplished,and published, a piece of written work – the completion of the task.

The writing process can constitute an important developmental learning experience in its own right. Working through a writing task from conception of an idea, through planning to crafting, editing and completion requires the author to demonstrate learning and a range of critical skills: not the least of which are organisation, synthesis and critique. The process of authoring requires all writers to clarify their thinking and develop their ability as communicators. But there are additional benefits of the writing process that may be achieved through collaboration with peers, either by co-authoring or peer reviewing. Checking with others that what you wish to say is worth saying, and that the way that you are saying it is clear, is both worthwhile and a common practice for many authors, from the novice through to the experienced writer. Colleagues may lend important insights and constructive criticism in relation to your work. And this process need not, of course, be confined to midwifery colleagues. There are often benefits to be had from working in broader professional and academic networks. In the academic context, this may entail collaboration with colleagues from other disciplines, other universities and even internationally. However, I am mindful of the danger of placing too much emphasis on the positive aspects of the process of writing. There is, of course, always a downside too! The writing process requires what is often a precious resource – time! And time to think, to plan and to execute the writing task rarely seems to be available in abundance. The benefits to the midwife of working through the writing process have, it always seems, to be carved out of an already over-committed day.

Yet, when this is possible and space to write does become available, authorship can bring a tremendous sense of achievement: I did that! I wrote that! Others felt that what I have to say is worth printing! Seeing a piece of written work that you have nurtured come out in print can give you a tremendous buzz! But, more than this, the midwife who is a published author assumes a public position with respect to ongoing debate and to knowledge generation. The published author has committed to an opinion; a stance; a perspective on the issue. They have put down a marker that, on an individual level, often forms an important element of individual assessment in institutional staff review and development appraisals. Publication may also help to position the individual, in a professional and an academic context, within a hierarchy of prestige.

There is clearly, therefore, benefit for the midwife author in the process of writing and in the outcome; in the completion of a writing task. However, the potential benefits of authorship do not only operate at the individual, personal level, but extend to the broader midwifery community and the midwifery profession as a whole. For the midwife in an academic role, a profile as a published author is protective of the academic department, both in terms of the professional presence and prestige that derives and through formal assessment of the quality of authorship that midwife academics may be subjected to – alongside colleagues in other areas of academia – as part of Research Assessment Exercises. The outcome of such assessments, which 'produce quality profiles for each submission of research activity made by institution(s)'[1], has direct implications for the financial well-being of departments in HE. In addition, authorship indicates and sustains a 'critical mass' of scholarship, evidencing a supportive research environment that may increase the success of future research funding applications and recruitment of research students and studentships.

Given the potential benefits of authorship, we need, therefore, to also consider the circumstances in which a midwife might choose not to write, recognising that the exercise of this responsibility may, at times, be uncomfortable. What the midwife has to say may be challenging to others. With my own unsuccessful writing experience outlined in the vignette, there was a singular failure to benefit the broader midwifery profession. In the face of opposition from experienced, well-respected colleagues, I failed to complete the writing process and did not submit the article I had drafted for publication. The opportunity to disseminate what I considered to be important messages about a practice innovation was not realised.

Reflecting on this experience led me to consider my own moral and/or ethical responsibility to write. My failure to complete the authoring process has crystallised into a strong belief that midwives do indeed have a moral and, often, ethical responsibility to write and to publish. By 'moral' responsibility, I assert that writing and publishing is the 'right' thing to do to encourage professional and public debate and to give voice to, and represent the experiences of, research participants. By 'ethical' responsibility, I refer to the requirement to adhere to principles of conduct that are generally considered to be correct (and that may be overseen and applied by research ethics committees); for example, that we should make clear which aspects of midwifery care have been determined to be effective – and, just as importantly – which aspects have not been so determined. This may not always be an easy responsibility to exercise, yet as members of a professional group with responsibility for client care, the onus falls upon us to foster dialogue, to enable reflexive consideration of all aspects of professional ethos and practice. Dialogue is not only good for midwifery, it is essential. The midwife author has the potential to extend the knowledge base for midwifery practice, to contribute to evidence-based care and, just as importantly, to strengthen theoretical understandings – for theory and practice must inform one another. Through authorship, the midwife disseminates research findings to a variety of user audiences, justifies and extends aspects of midwifery practice and challenges others. There should be no no-go areas. If we cannot write about, discuss and critique any aspect of midwifery practice, this probably means that we cannot justify it. A profession that fears to air or acknowledge its own limitations surely threatens to undermine its own foundations and the basis for its independent existence.

Midwives have, therefore, a moral and ethical obligation to write; to open up to scrutiny and debate (both professional and public) accepted ways of understanding, assumptions and practices. However, authorship may also be a two-edged sword, for the pressure to publish, especially for the midwife in an academic role, is persistent and increasing.

Some reflections on the practice of writing

Although the curriculum in English schools currently emphasises the different writing styles that are required for different forms of communication, I suspect that many of us have reached adulthood with limited preparation for many aspects of writing. On the whole, no one teaches us how to write and authorship can invoke an uncomfortable feeling of insecurity. Mastering academic writing, in particular, may seem like mastering a foreign language: any midwife academic will readily describe the tendency for students to obscure what they are trying to say through the use of (what the student deems to be) 'academic' vocabulary.

There are always, of course, colleagues who write fluidly, cogently and apparently spontaneously. To those of us who are less fortunate, the practice of writing can perhaps more accurately be described as 'like pulling teeth'. Writing, as the American novelist Paul Theroux is reputed to have said, 'is pretty crummy on the nerves'.[2]

There is a wealth of advice available to the budding author in books, online resources and writing for publication courses. These provide advice and suggest techniques for organising, writing and editing the writing project and some suggestions for further reading are included in Box 15.1.

Although there is no intention to summarise the available advice here, some aspects of the practice of writing are worth commenting upon – though in doing so I acknowledge that these are firmly

---

Box 15.1

There is a wealth of advice available. See, for example:

Books

Cook, R. and Norman, A. (1999) *The Writer's Manual: A step-by-step guide for nurses and other health professionals*, Oxford: Radcliffe Publishing.

Henson, K.T. (2004) *Writing for Publication: Road to academic advancement*, Needham Heights, MA: Pearson/Allyn & Bacon.

Johnstone, M.-J. (2004) *Effective Writing for Health Professionals: A practical guide to getting published*, London and New York: Routledge.

Oermann, M.H. (2005) *Writing for Publication in Nursing*, Philadelphia, PA: Lippincott Williams & Wilkins.

Sigismund Huff, A. (1998) *Writing for Scholarly Publication*, London: Sage.

Journal articles

These include guidance and/or discussion about the writing and the publication process:

Dixon, N. (2001) 'Writing for publication: a guide for new authors', *International Journal for Quality in Health Care* 13(5): 417–21.

Happell, B. (2005) 'Disseminating nursing knowledge: a guide to writing for publication', *International Journal of Psychiatric Nursing Research* 10(3): 1147–55.

Happell, B. (2008) 'Writing for publication: a practical guide', *Nursing Standard* 22(28): 35–40.

Keen, A. (2007) 'Writing for publication: pressures, barriers and support strategies', *Nurse Education Today* 27(5): 382–8.

Miracle, V.A. (2003) 'Writing for publication: you can do it!', *Dimensions of Critical Care Nursing* 22(1): 31–4.

Thomson, A.M. (2005) 'Writing for publication in this refereed journal', *Midwifery* 21(2): 190–4.

embedded in my specific experiences and other authors may well have generated a very different emphasis:

- There may only be a subtle distinction, at times, between 'drafting' and 'writing', but approaching a writing task as a draft can liberate the author to think about *what* they want to say rather than just *how* they want to say it.
- Organisation is key: writing often requires reorganisation, editing, further reorganisation, further editing . . . and so on.
- It is as important for an author to decide what to keep out of their writing project as it is to decide what to put in.
- If you get lost, and find yourself easily distracted from your writing task, look carefully at your organisation. Are you clear about what you are trying to say?
- If you are really getting nowhere and feel as if you're going round in circles, take a break and come back with fresh eyes in a few hours or days or even weeks.

With my own writing, I struggle with organisation and am easily sidetracked. I have spent, over the years, what must amount to several days looking through the thesaurus for a precise word in order to craft a sentence. Eventually, I have come to accept that this is nothing more than a distraction, taking me away from the task of writing. However, even with acceptance, I still find myself doing this on occasions. For example, while writing this chapter I chose to look up the meaning of the word 'process' in online dictionaries. Process is a word that I use frequently and have little difficulty with. I did come across a new word – 'obviousism', which I am informed means 'an expression of obviousness',[3] but this has been of little use to me other than to illustrate how easy it is to distract myself from the task of writing! The majority of authors probably have their own foibles. What matters is that, where a midwife occupies a role that requires them to write, there is a need to reflect upon the challenges experienced and explore ways of managing these.

Some reflections on the process of getting published

Some midwives, and particularly those working in the HE sector, are subject to persistent and increasing pressure to publish. The moral and ethical issues that I perceived in relation to my failure to publish were, in reality, only part of the picture: I also feared the loss of a publication opportunity.

Moreover, the pressure on individuals within HE to publish is increasingly influenced by institutional considerations, rather than the needs of practitioners or of the broader user community. The academic midwife has to balance, on the one hand, a responsibility to practice colleagues and to the families of childbearing women and, on the other hand, the increasing pressure, evident within the HE sector, to target publications in light of externally defined quality criteria. As new forms of Research Assessment are introduced in the university sector, it is likely that this balance will be skewed increasingly in favour of journals that assume greatest significance in journal citation indexes,[4] rather than those most accessible to practitioners and other parts of the user communities.

Midwives working outside the HE sector may experience different pressures upon them to prioritise particular forms of dissemination and publication. Ideally, however, decisions about how to craft a writing project for publication should be made only after carefully considering a range of questions, some of which are highlighted in Box 15.2.

Although by no means exhaustive, these are suggestive of some of the questions an author might consider as they commit to a writing project and work towards getting published. The way in which an individual responds to these will vary over time and between projects; however, there are some considerations to be mindful of: writing for different audiences often requires different presentational styles. Journals that concentrate on the audience that you intend to target will have a 'house–style' that they deem to be effective as a means of communicating with their readership. The potential author may only get a feel for this style by identifying and carefully reading articles that have some similarity to the article under preparation. Familiarisation with this house style is different from, though no less important than, a thorough understanding of the guidance to authors that all journals provide. The latter clarifies key presentational elements expected for all submissions and should not be ignored. If a prospective author is unclear about whether a specific journal is an appropriate outlet for a writing project, having read the journal's aims and reviewed some of the articles already published, an enquiry directed at the editor is often possible. Once you are clear that you have targeted an appropriate outlet, submission is now usually achieved by means of what can seem to be a complex, online

---

Box 15.2

- Have you got something new/different to say?
- Who do you want to read your work? Why should they?
- Where might you publish to make your work available to them?
- What is the most appropriate format?
- Do you know enough about your proposed publication medium (for example, the aims and target audience of a journal)?
- What sort of balance between academic/accessible language will best suit your target audience? Is this compatible with your intended publication medium?
- Can you write enough words for the medium (for example, the journal article) that you have in mind? Or can you say what you need to within the word constraints?
- Do you need your publication to carry with it other 'values' (for example, does it need to be a peer-reviewed article)?
- Does it need to be in a journal that ranks highly in the citation indexes?
- Will your message still be current by the time others get to see it (for example, by the time it gets through the publication cycle)?

---

submission system. From this point, several weeks of waiting can be expected, which may stretch into months for the more prestigious journals, before authors receive feedback on their submissions.

One of the key techniques for quality assurance in the publication process is the use of anonymous refereeing of submitted articles. This means that the writing project that you submit will be independently reviewed – often by two or more anonymous reviewers who are members either of the editorial board or of a much larger panel of reviewers who have expertise in the subject area. These reviewers will make recommendations to the editor about the quality of your submission and its suitability for publication. For some, the process ends at this point with rejection by the journal. This decision is absolute and final and the author is left with only two possible courses of action: to discard the piece of work and move on, or to re-submit to a different journal.

Having an article accepted for publication without the requirement to undertake amendments is a rare experience. More frequently, authors receive anonymous (and even, sometimes, contradictory) comments from the reviewers and an invitation to re-submit a revised paper. This can be a challenging time for authors, and the idea of undertaking substantial work on a writing project that had been completed and 'ticked off' can seem overwhelming. After the initial, perhaps inevitable, disappointment and the benefit of reflection, reviewers' comments are usually insightful, constructive and aimed at improving – rather than destroying – the piece of work. However, it is important to recognise, at this stage, that amending an article in a manner that takes into consideration the comments of the reviewers does not guarantee that it will subsequently be accepted for publication: rejection remains a real possibility.

For authors who successfully negotiate the publication process and whose articles are accepted by a journal, further delays are then encountered as the paper goes through the process of being formatted and prepared for print. After a long period of inactivity, a final effort is required from the author, who must confirm the accuracy of the formatted paper before it goes into the journal's queue for publication. Online journals and those that have online availability in advance of a printed copy may only have a short delay before the author can access their published output. However, a hard copy may still be many months away. The length of the publication cycle varies considerably between journals, but it is often a long and a slow process. As Ann Thomson has noted, 'Acceptance of a paper for publication sometimes appears to be a mountain that has to be climbed.'[5]

Conclusion

Authorship is fundamental to the credibility and development of the midwifery profession. Differently positioned midwives may experience authorship as a moral and ethical responsibility to varying degrees, although a common factor in the experience of many is a lack of proactive support to enable the ongoing development of confidence, as a writer, and skill as a communicator through the medium of the written word.

For midwives to write effectively they must know what they want to say, why it is worth saying and how it relates to the existing knowledge base. Although writing can be highly pressured, and is not without its challenges, it can also be highly rewarding and an aspect of midwifery practice that we ignore at our peril.

Commentary

Penny's sad vignette and the reflection arising out of it takes us way beyond the usual 'how to' approach of publication manuals. These manuals often do little more than enhance editorial power and limit that of the author by conventions such as submission to just one journal at a time.[6] The valuable insights that Penny shares with us lend a new meaning to writing; and this meaning will be new even to experienced writers.

This reflection on writing is novel, adopting as it does the viewpoint of both the individual midwife and the midwifery profession as a whole. The reason for this is because writing tends to be quite a solitary activity. Although there may be collaborators checking drafts and contributing different parts of the 'finished product', the individual author needs peace and quiet in order to make progress.

This need for peace echoes what Penny writes about the distractions that she encounters. Thanks to Penny, I will now see my thesaurus in a completely new light. Rather than being a friend and ally, Penny seems to have converted it into a menace, which now threatens to impede my productivity!

More seriously, though, Penny explains the nature of distractions in terms of their being problematical. It may be that there is something else going on for Penny, when she is waylaid by her thesaurus. Perhaps this is her way of taking a little 'time out' from her writing task. It may be that she has reached the point of feeling that she is 'brain dead' and the spark of ideas is elusive. So her time spent with her thesaurus may be a fairly constructive way to take a break. This may allow her time to replenish her batteries of ideas. It may even mean that there is some degree of subliminal reflection happening during her communication with her thesaurus. This is the way that I rationalise the 'time out' that I spend doing the relatively mind-numbing tasks, such as checking the word count and getting the references into the correct format.

Importantly, Penny writes about the need for dialogue within midwifery. I would like to build on her argument, by suggesting that dialogue is also needed between midwife authors and their readers. Although, very occasionally, midwifery journals feature correspondence on news items, rarely does this include a response to a published paper. This may be because midwives are nice people, but I would argue that midwife authors deserve and need this form of feedback. This form of communication is being used in preparing this book to encourage 'conversation' between the authors and the editors. It should be used more widely if the knowledge base on which midwifery is founded is to become as authoritative as the profession deserves.

Notes

1   Online at www.rae.ac.uk (accessed 8 September 2009).
2   Online at www.great-quotes.com/cgi-bin/viewquotes.cgi?action=search &Author_First_Name=Paul&Author_Last_Name=Theroux&Movie= (accessed 7 May 2009).
3   *Merriam Webster Open Dictionary*: obviousism (noun): an expression of obviousness: 'The client's case was full of obviousism and winning would be easy.' Online at www3.merriam-webster.com/opendictionary/ newword_display_recent.php?id=41526 (accessed 7 May 2009).
4   For example, *Journal Citation Reports*®, which is defined by Thomson Reuters as follows:

The recognized authority for evaluating journals, *Journal Citation Reports* presents quantifiable statistical data that provides a systematic, objective way to evaluate the world's leading journals and their impact and influence in the global research community.

Online at http://scientific.thomsonreuters.com/products/jcr/ (accessed 21 July 2008).
5   Thomson, A.M. (2005) 'Writing for publication in this refereed journal', *Midwifery* 21(2): 190–4. Quote from p. 190.
6   Mander, R. (2009) 'Publishing issues', *MIDIRS* 18(4): 471–3.

Chapter 16

The ex-midwife

Elaine Haycock-Stuart

Introduction

In this chapter, I reflect on why I entered midwifery and on my recollections of how I experienced midwifery in the late 1980s. Following on from this reflection, I utilise a vignette to illustrate why I became an ex-midwife.

How it all began

Why did I decide to become a midwife and then an ex-midwife or, rather, a health visitor? I decided at a young age (about 7 years) that nursing was the job I wanted to do and I owe much of my continuing desire to nurse to my parents, who supported this interest and enthusiasm! There is no family history of the caring professions, yet they valued my choices and respected the work nurses and midwives do. As a child, I was given opportunities to attend the Red Cross and develop first aid skills, alongside other useful things, such as lifesaving skills with swimming. At 16 I undertook work experience with my school, where I was encouraged to look at alternatives to nursing and spent two weeks working in a pathology laboratory in the local district hospital. It was enough time for me to be sure that laboratory work was not for me! I recognised that I enjoyed the interpersonal aspects of life, despite being shy, and that a more communicative, humanising experience was important to me. At sixth-form college, it was generally accepted that I had decided to nurse and that was that; there was no careers advice! I was eager to nurse and my family supported the decision.

Nursing

I undertook my nursing education in a large city hospital in the north of England about 90 minutes away from my home. Initially, it took time for me to adapt to being away from home, but eventually I made some great friends (we have recently had a 25-year reunion). I found nursing academically stimulating, yet it was emotionally draining on many occasions. For example, aged 18, I had to nurse a young girl who was also 18 years old, in a coma following a road traffic accident. Her A level results came through and she had three straight As! Such sadness and heartbreak for the family. I felt that this side of nursing work was emotionally draining, but that being able to care for such ill individuals and supporting their families was a valuable role.

As a nurse, I found myself being attacked in the hospital wards by men who were in a state of confusion post-myocardial infarction; one hurled a fire extinguisher at me! It was the humour of the other patients and my co-students that got me through much of the turmoil. There was not always a funny side to everything, but, when there was, it was important to see it. I was a good hospital nurse, so I am told. I even won a prize or two, but in my nursing programme I enjoyed my community midwifery and health visiting experience and felt that this was where I would like to focus my career.

I made the decision that the 'real world' was where I wanted to work, not in the hospital environment. I enjoyed meeting and speaking with people on their terms – usually in their own homes or occasionally at the GP surgery. I made plans for further education to become a health visitor, but several people I spoke to, both health visitors and nurses, advised me to gain experience as a midwife before considering health visiting. I respected this advice as it came from several experienced people, so I applied for midwifery education. I was successful in obtaining a place in the same hospital where I had become a nurse.

Becoming a midwife

The nursing and midwifery programmes were worlds apart! I had enjoyed my nursing course, but loved my midwifery course. I was not just stimulated, I was challenged. The integration of theory and practice, the clinical rotations – it was very lively and 'happening'. I really had to stay on top of the academic work, which was assessed every couple of weeks by class exam. I had to integrate my theory knowledge daily with my clinical practice and be prepared to move every few weeks to a different clinical area of midwifery – labour ward, antenatal ward, postnatal ward, community and neonatal high dependency! It was a fantastic time.

The things I value

Midwifery's strength, in my view, lies in its focus on the mother and newborn baby – the specificity of the midwifery work with women during pregnancy, during birth, and immediately after, enables midwives to become knowledgeable and skilled in great depth. I considered myself and other midwives to have relatively narrow but deep knowledge and skills as the work is so focused, as opposed to the broad and superficial knowledge and skills that I associate with other areas of nursing. As a midwife, I felt I knew a great deal about caring for maternal health during pregnancy and labour, and postnatally, in addition to foetal development and care of the newborn baby up to 28 days. This clarity of role and function was and still is, to me, one of the best things about midwifery work compared with other areas of nursing.

Reflecting on nursing and particularly midwifery, I am usually drawn to the sensational, rarer, significant events, as these seem to make up most of my memories from my midwifery career. The more regular and everyday experiences are less remarkable, but not in any way mundane. However, these daily experiences do not form my main reflections on midwifery; it is often the more remarkable events that I dwell on. For this reason, I will reflect on midwifery the way I see it, through the sensational, more than the routine. This is not necessarily how other working midwives would describe or reflect on their current work.

Sensational times

Below, I give some reflections on being involved in midwifery care; I have mentioned how difficult it is to do this in an unbiased way and how easy it is to be drawn to the sensational. It is also important to appreciate that, as an ex-midwife, I am describing a dynamic profession and my reflections are on service in the late 1980s and early 1990s. I know there are similarities with the current context, but there are also vast differences and what I am reflecting on is not necessarily how it is today.

New Year's Eve, night shift and the delivery suite (labour ward) is frantically busy with women in labour and family members providing support. I am supporting a couple expecting their first baby; the wife is in the throws of delivery. I am prepared for the arrival of a new baby when the father faints and bangs his head on the floor – the accident book will have to wait! The mother is the one who needs supporting with this delivery! The father will have to take second place. Happily a 'normal' delivery, no complications – except I have to complete the accident book for the father, who now has a big bump on his head!

Half an hour later and minutes from midnight and I am supporting a couple expecting their first baby – the father has declared he has no desire to be present at the actual birth. I cannot find another member of staff who is not completely involved in a delivery elsewhere – no midwife, no auxiliary, no student! I need a hand; this is a big baby – the mother is tall, but when all is said and done, this is a BIG baby. I ask the dad just to give a hand as much as he can. Gently, he is coaxed by the mother and me to help support her through the delivery, helping her with her breathing, supporting and massaging her back. Thankfully he is looking less stressed and more like he might start to enjoy being at the delivery – I reassure him that I am hopeful I will have help from a colleague at the actual birth. The progress is fast – the baby is ready to be delivered and we are just after midnight! We might get the first New Year's Day baby!! (Every year we have a 'little competition' between the other city hospital and ourselves as to which will have the first baby of the year!) Not going too smoothly – this baby is big, the head has crowned, but there is shoulder dystocia (the upper body is more difficult to deliver) and the clock is ticking. Sister pops her head round. 'Can I give a hand?' she asks. Our eyes meet and she comes straight in to help. 'Come on baby, come on baby, come!' Thankfully, this ten-pound baby has a safe, normal delivery. Even dad is looking happy. It turns out we didn't get the first baby of the year though! Time for a cup of tea I think.

It is not so long before a mother who is in labour with her third child (she has two children that she delivered normally) arrives with her husband. Third baby – this indicates she could be progressing fast and be ready to deliver. I examine the mother and listen to the foetal heart – the baby's heart rate is slow – much too slow at 45 beats per minute! (A normal heart rate is in the range of 120–160 beats per minute depending on the level of the foetal activity.) I ask the mother to turn on to her side and explain that she and the baby would benefit from a little oxygen. They are a very calm couple and I am grateful for that. The oxygen has made no difference – the heart rate is very slow. I excuse myself from the couple for a few minutes and go directly to sister. Calmly, I explain quietly about what I have assessed and the actions I have taken. 'Are you certain it is the foetal heart and not the maternal pulse you are listening to? Have you given her oxygen?' she asks as we both walk back to the couple. We both know this is serious and my recording the maternal pulse in error, instead of the baby's, would be something of a relief as it would indicate the baby is in better shape than I think it is. But I know I have made no error and that the maternal pulse is actually faster than the baby's – this woman needs to be in theatre right now and there is no theatre available. I had hoped a third baby would be a lovely, straightforward, normal delivery without too long to wait. This is not going to happen. Sister examines the woman and listens to the baby's heart rate. She speaks reassuringly to the couple, but explains that this baby needs to be delivered in theatre. Sister stays with the couple as I head to prepare for theatre – we usually act as scrub nurses for our own operative deliveries. I speak to the senior registrar in theatre and let him know that we have a very urgent need for him to be ready to move straight on to another Caesarean section. I explain the circumstances to him and he acknowledges the urgency of the situation. He is rapidly outside assessing the mother and within minutes she is in theatre. The husband has to wait patiently outside, as this is an emergency section – not planned and we sense there is a complication. The baby is delivered gently – the cord is wrapped around the neck twice! The baby would not have survived a normal delivery. Mother and baby are both well.

Here I am reflecting on the sensational, but this is very much the reality of life in the labour ward. Yes, there is a great deal of monitoring and waiting, but it is an exciting and stressful place to work, too. No two days are the same, but I did have some days when I did not deliver a baby and spent a great deal of time monitoring and supporting women only for them to deliver on the next shift. This could be disappointing, but I enjoyed supporting women in labour, too, and other days could see me delivering two or three babies.

What is it all about?

Here I offer some reflections on my observations of acute-setting midwifery within different contexts and environments. These show the kinds of things that I was involved with in midwifery, although I do not feel I had many 'typical' days, as most were quite special.

Labour ward

The work in the labour ward could be diverse, for example supporting or ensuring smooth running in theatre for a woman having a Caesarean section, delivering a baby for a woman having a normal delivery or monitoring a woman in early labour. Occasionally, a woman may need support delivering a stillborn baby or a doctor may need the midwife to assist with a forceps or complicated delivery and support the woman. There is a great variety in how women labour and in the nature of support they and their families need.

They say variety is the spice of life and I feel this is particularly true for me when I worked in the labour ward or delivery suite. For me, every delivery was different – the dynamics of very different women and partners make it so. Then you have the different ways people 'progress' during labour and how they eventually deliver the baby and the responses they have to a new baby, as well as the different health outcomes of each new baby at delivery. Many factors influence this very dynamic process in the labour ward and there is really very little that I, on reflection, would call 'typical' about it.

Antenatal ward

Some women may be in the antenatal ward to rest, to be monitored, or to have further investigations for the management of a complicated pregnancy, such as a low-lying placenta. Some may be in the ward in advance of a planned Caesarean section for a breech baby, while others may be hospitalised as a result of an illness, such as unstable diabetes, or may require specific nursing care in relation to a medical condition. As a midwife, I would be caring for women with very different needs and some women would spend a considerable length of time within the ward, whereas others might only be there a day or two. Some women would require high levels of nursing and personal care and others might be closely monitored but independent.

Many women in antenatal wards are concerned about other dependants and family members at home and rarely are women in the antenatal ward happy to be there! In my experience, some women were resident for lengthy periods and were unhappy about their hospitalisation; they often felt well in themselves and they really wanted to be home. I often had the feeling that the antenatal ward had parallels with a prison for some women and that they hoped for the 'great escape'. Often as a midwife I felt I was viewed more as a jailer by some women – encouraging them to rest – than as a supportive midwife. The women wanted to be home with their families and my observation of them and their foetus was all that prevented them from escaping!

An interesting observation about midwives and antenatal wards is that, although midwives normally only conduct normal deliveries, every woman on an antenatal ward has a potentially complicated delivery. I always find this something of a paradox! Midwives need to know such a great deal about 'abnormal' pregnancy, but usually only conduct deliveries that are normal – admittedly they give support to complicated births too! As a midwife on an antenatal ward, I felt that most of the women I was caring for were unlikely to have a normal delivery – yet I undertook a great deal of antenatal care with them. When these women did come to deliver, it was often a labour ward midwife who would be present at the delivery to support the woman and the doctor, not usually the midwife who had cared for her during a lengthy antenatal ward stay. This was often disappointing for the mothers and the antenatal ward midwives who had developed trusting, caring relationships. Arguably, during a complicated delivery the antenatal midwife should be better able to support mothers they have cared for.

Postnatal ward

Work on the postnatal ward involved helping mothers wishing to breastfeed and to develop bonding strategies and childcare skills, for example feeding, bathing, changing and bonding through touch, eye contact and singing. I would help prepare the mothers for caring for themselves and their babies independently on discharge. I would examine the mothers and their babies to ensure everything was normal.

The postnatal ward is usually a happy place, but sometimes people have complicated deliveries or babies become unwell and this requires the midwife to be skilful in their observations and communications with mothers and families. Mothers can also feel quite low after the delivery, yet feel they are under family or peer pressure to be happy at the new birth. Some parents struggle to adapt in the early days to caring for a new baby and sometimes babies are 'unwanted' or are to be adopted. The postnatal environment is complex and no assumptions should be made about how women feel and respond to babies after childbirth, as this is a very personal experience and requires the skills of observation and sensitivity on the part of midwives to support mothers after delivery.

It is late evening as we come towards the end of a late shift and I am in the nursery on the postnatal ward talking with the two nursery nurses who have worked here for many years. As we feed and change babies whose mums are resting, one asks me about my decision to leave midwifery. 'Why are you going?' Earlier in the week, I had informed the ward staff that I would be going to study to become a health visitor in the autumn. It seems it came as a great surprise to staff; the senior house officer had said to me, 'You are the last person I would have expected to leave! You are so together here!'

In truth I am a little uncertain about my decision. I came into midwifery with the ultimate aim of becoming a health visitor. I have enjoyed my midwifery education and staffing immensely, and I have stayed longer than I needed, but I have really enjoyed it so much that I did not envisage leaving to become a health visitor again until I moved to Scotland. Should I let a few frustrations force me out? Are they just a few frustrations or are they really something quite big and problematic?

I came to Scotland and took a while to adjust to the climate, but that was not the only reason for me often feeling low in those first few months. At work, when I first arrived, I was handed a cardboard box and informed that it was the resuscitation equipment for the babies! I was mortified – this was primitive! On a subsequent occasion, I asked about gloves for examining the mothers and babies – none were supplied and, when I started ordering them, I was reprimanded for the cost implication. I was working in a city with high rates of HIV, but I seemed to be the only person concerned about the midwives' welfare with regard to the transmission of infection.

I started taking blood when it was required by the doctors (I had been trained to do this down south), and again I was reprimanded – 'Midwives do not do that on this ward'! When I did take blood, I had to draw it up by syringe and squirt it into containers. I had been used to the syringes with needles that snapped off – syringes that were sent to the laboratory for investigation, in order to reduce spillage of blood and transmissions of infection. Several things made me feel I had stepped back in time ten years!! (*Life on Mars: The midwifery story?* Perhaps not!) Eventually, I was asked to help teach some of the other midwives and students how to take blood – it was good to see progress.

I have asked several times to be allowed to rotate to a different clinical area during my year here on the postnatal ward, but this has not been granted and I have been advised that it would be a considerable length of time before I could expect to move to another area. Occasionally, I have been moved briefly to help in a different clinical area if they were short-staffed, but this has been rare. Are these good reasons for moving on? I think so and I explain to the nursery nurses why, for these kinds of reasons, I am going.

'It's a big shame for us – we will be sad to see you go,' they reply. I am surprised by their comment and I ask them why? They explain to me their observations – apparently I am the only staff midwife who allocates myself mothers and babies when I am in charge of the ward, so it evens out the workload. The other staff midwives take no mothers or babies, but stick with managerial work only, for example the ward round and medicine round. I had never noticed this, but it matters to the nursery nurses – to them it shows I care about the clinical care, not purely management. It also shows I share the work more equitably. It seems many of my colleagues are not continuing with hands-on clinical contact with mothers and babies when they are in charge – I wonder why this should be so? I know being in charge has managerial commitments, but I always combine these with clinical work. Sometimes I ask colleagues to keep a close eye on my mothers and babies for a brief time if I am involved heavily in a managerial aspect of work, but I do not absolve myself from clinical responsibilities and clearly my junior colleagues value this approach. This just reaffirms to me that I need to move on. I do not want to start adopting the same purely managerial approach to my work. I enjoy working with the mothers, but really do not enjoy the constraints on my professional sphere of practice and future professional development. I have made the right decision – I think?

Looking back

Initially, as a qualified midwife, my work was diverse and the three-monthly rotations in the first city hospital I worked in meant I felt capable of moving into different clinical areas of midwifery with relative ease and little anxiety – we would rotate through the labour ward and antenatal/postnatal wards about every 12 weeks. A typical day is hard to define, as each area was so very different – a typical day in the labour ward was not the same as a typical day in and antenatal or postnatal ward. Variety and change were brilliant and I think form one of the strengths of midwifery. I had less opportunity to rotate through clinical areas when I moved to Scotland and spent a year in the postnatal ward. I considered this deskilling and was frustrated at, among other things, the lack of opportunity to rotate through the clinical areas – and this was a main driver for me moving out of midwifery and into health visiting. I had primarily entered midwifery in preparation for becoming a midwife and I turned to health visiting when I became dissatisfied with the organisational infrastructure for midwifery in the hospital I worked in.

Was health visiting a good choice?

In truth, midwifery and health visiting are worlds apart and it would take a further chapter – possibly a book – to reflect fully on my experiences of both, but midwifery was valuable within my subsequent work as a health visitor. I am not convinced midwifery is essential in becoming a health visitor, as many people had led me to believe. There are aspects of midwifery that, without a doubt, have helped me in my subsequent work as a health visitor, but there is much more it did not prepare me for. Health visiting, too, has evolved dramatically in the last 18 years and, in reality, the work now is different from when I first started – child protection is now a main feature of health visiting work and midwifery does not prepare you well for this. I eventually left health visiting and clinical practice following doctoral studies as there was, and still is, a lack of opportunity for clinical research careers – despite the rhetoric and the policy development in this area. I am now a Senior Lecturer, using my nursing, midwifery and health visiting experience in an academic research career.

Conclusion

I enjoyed midwifery in both the hospital and the community and worked a variety of shifts, for example evenings, nights and mornings. There are now assessment units for midwives to use their skills further. Midwifery work is varied, interesting and valuable; it is a dynamic environment in which I learned to enjoy 'change', which I think has been of great benefit to me in my subsequent career.

My reflections beg the question – why would you want to leave something you enjoyed so much? There are a few reasons and all are related to the organisation of midwifery in the late 1980s and are not necessarily the same now. For me, midwifery needs regular rotation, not necessarily every 12 weeks, but at least every 6 months. I was unable to be guaranteed a rotation of any kind when I moved to Scotland. Some of the extended roles I undertook in England were not permitted in Scotland at the time and I felt I was being deskilled. Promotion within midwifery looked limited and, although I did not realise it at the time, I was ambitious. I began to feel midwifery was shrinking around me as I became limited to the postnatal clinical area, inhibited in the clinical skills I could practise, and saw promotion as a very distant point on a very long horizon.

I enjoyed the work, but needed the variety that I had enjoyed earlier in my midwifery career.

I always say I would go back to midwifery given half a chance, because I remember it fondly, enjoyed it and valued the work I did. I love the clear-cut focus of the remit of the midwife, with the vast opportunity for variety within that focus. So what holds me back? Today, it is still to some extent the reasons given above, but in addition there is the more personal impact of how midwifery is organised – where is the good 24/7 childcare that women in the caring professions need in order to work shifts when they have no family support living near by? As a mother of a young child, with a partner who works abroad a great deal of time and no family within 240 miles, I could not return to shift work without flexible 24/7 childcare. Midwifery and, indeed, nursing are female-dominated professions and there needs to be more consideration of family-friendly policies. In the future, many of us will be caring for elderly family members, so if we are not caring for children we will probably be looking after an older person. If the NHS addressed these issues, maybe I would be less of an ex and more of a midwife!

Commentary

Elaine's chapter shows very clearly that being a midwife is a lifelong commitment and that this even applies to the midwife who is no longer practising as such. The discomfort or dissonance that she experienced around the time of her decision to leave midwifery is all too apparent.

The mention by Elaine of providing nursing care for an 18 year old reminds us that we have so much in common with those for whom we provide care. These commonalities may present themselves quite suddenly and unexpectedly. This may cause uncomfortable feelings of 'What is different?' and 'What is similar?' These common or shared feelings may threaten the boundaries within which we ordinarily work quite comfortably; by this I mean my knowing who I am and my certainty about the role that I am fulfilling.

These boundaries, which may be summarised as separating our professional and personal selves, emerged in a research project I undertook (Mander 2004). Effectively, the midwives in this study told me of their pain at being forced to confront their own humanity in a challenging situation. The midwives who spoke to me were able to find good support to help them through the experience, and many contacted their supervisor of midwives (see Chapter 7). So midwives' support for each other may be very effective, but sometimes it is less so (see Chapter 12).

It was a source of regret to Elaine that she was not able to offer good continuity of care to the women for whom she cared in the antenatal ward. Since Elaine was practising, 'continuity' has become something of a cliché. This development was associated with the publication of the report, *Changing Childbirth* (DH 1993). Although this report attracted considerable publicity and may have caused the care providers to contemplate the services provided for childbearing women, it is necessary to question whether the standard of care has really been changed. It may be that, to midwives, as was stated by nursing's icon, Florence Nightingale, 'Reports are not self-executive'.

Of particular importance to midwives is the issue that Elaine raises about family-friendly policies in the health care system. Although we tend to assume that this means child-friendly, Elaine reminds us that it may also apply to the midwife caring for an elderly dependant. Because midwifery is such a largely female occupational group and because caring roles still tend to be assumed by the mother, wife or daughter, family friendliness or, rather, the lack of it is a source of concern to many who work in health care. It may be necessary, like Elaine, to question how many ex-midwives would still be practising midwives were genuinely family-friendly arrangements in place.

References

Department of Health (DH) (1993) *Changing Childbirth*, Report of The Expert Maternity Group, London: HMSO.

Mander, R. (2004) 'When the professional gets personal: the midwife's experience of the death of a mother', *Evidence-based Midwifery* 2: 240–5.

Conclusion

Rosemary Mander and Valerie Fleming

As we mentioned in the Introduction to this book, the intention was to provide material for two groups of people. These groups comprise people contemplating midwifery, either as a new or a continuing career. The contributors have explored a host of different aspects of the midwifery role. Many of these aspects have shown midwifery for what it is – a truly wonderful opportunity to make a difference to people's lives. I hope, though, that this book has shown midwifery to be something more than that. It involves amazingly complex social, professional and human situations. It may be necessary for you, the reader, to decide whether and to what extent this reality accords with your aspirations.

The issues that have been raised have provided a wealth of food for thought. On the basis of these issues, the potential or actual midwife is able to contemplate her or his career. Additionally, it is clear that these issues affect all concerned with women's health in general and with the maternity services in particular.

Issues emerging

These issues present a complex picture of a far from straightforward professional group. In some ways, the authors have presented a picture of a job that may seem well-nigh perfect. This is apparent in Chapter 8, which explores how some people may see the role of the academic midwife. Similarly, Ans in Chapter 9 suggests that being a midwife researcher may be regarded as quite idyllic. In these two chapters, as in others, the focus moves on to the reality of what the midwife does; this may differ from these first impressions.

An aspect of midwifery that has resonated loud and clear throughout the pages of this book is its dynamism. Particularly significant, as shown by Yvonne in Chapter 1, is the dynamic nature of the relationship between the midwife and both the childbearing woman and the other disciplines who contribute to her care. Eleanor shows, through her innovations outlined in Chapter 4, how practice is changing. In her commentary on Chapter 8, on the academic midwife, Valerie emphasises the crucial nature of education in bringing about change. Lindsay's contribution on the midwife historian, Chapter 10, shows how changes happen in midwifery, and the extent to which fashions come and go. This chapter also helps us to contemplate the way that future developments may unfold. But this future may also be a source of concern. This anxiety may arise out of Nessa's account in Chapter 12 of what is happening to the independent midwife. In the same way, the exciting prospects proposed by *Changing Childbirth* (DH 1993), such as the continuity of care(r) raised by Elaine in Chapter 16, may not have been completely realised.

Particularly encouraging is the way that the authors have shown that certain neglected or 'Cinderella' areas of midwifery practice are at long last being given the attention, by practitioners and researchers, that they both need and deserve. Such areas include the perinatal mental health problems discussed by Eleanor in Chapter 4. The same may be said to apply to the management issues in midwifery explored by Georgina in Chapter 5. Allison, in writing about care of the mother and baby at home in Chapter 3, explicitly states that community postnatal care has been regarded as one of the Cinderella services. We may argue that the provision of postnatal care is increasingly recognised as crucially important. It may be that these areas have for far too long been neglected because they are not as exciting, or perhaps as 'sexy', as the high-profile, attention-grabbing areas of antenatal care or care in labour.

Another aspect of midwifery that may be beginning to attract some much-needed attention is the human or humane side of what midwives do and how midwives are affected by what they do. In Chapter 5, when she writes about being a midwife manager, Georgina considers the context of midwifery and how seriously the social aspects impinge on the midwives and their managers. In writing about the role of the supervisor of midwives in Chapter 7, Jean demonstrates the humanity of this role by showing that it is fundamentally all about supporting the practitioner. The independent midwife, as described by Nessa in Chapter 12, may be particularly in need of support. Nessa shows that, although this support works well when it does work, there may be times when support is not forthcoming. Writing as an ex-midwife in Chapter 16, Elaine discusses some of the personal and social aspects of being a midwife.

She goes on to explain, though, that the lack of what are now called 'family-friendly policies' played a large part in her decision to move out of midwifery. The human aspects of being a midwifery student are addressed by Elma in her consideration in Chapter 6 of the midwife as mentor.

Another important issue that emerged, as it so often does, is the extent to which midwifery is a profession. In Chapter 15, writing about the midwife author, Penny argues the need for more professional dialogue within midwifery. Miranda, in Chapter 2 on the midwife practising in a labour ward setting, touches on the professional issues. These arise out of Miranda's splendid account of this midwife being an expert in multi-skilling and multi-tasking. Such wide-ranging expertise may cause you, the reader, to wonder whether and to what extent this role fits into the more traditional definitions of a profession. Similarly, throughout Chapter 5, Georgina discusses midwifery in terms of a service to be provided. This service role may not fit very comfortably with the professional ethos.

Not unrelated to the professional debate is the relationship between the midwife and those with or alongside whom he or she practises. The relationship with colleagues emerges in Chapter 4, when Eleanor emphasises the fundamental importance of teamwork in perinatal mental health care. The relationship between the midwife and the childbearing woman emerges even more frequently. This is raised by Georgina, the midwife manager, in Chapter 5, when she contemplates the woman's input into the maternity services and the extent to which this may constitute a partnership. This relationship also appears in Chapter 9, by Ans, on the midwife researcher, when we are reminded that the ultimate purpose of research is to benefit the childbearing woman. In Chapter 14, this relationship re-emerges through the exploration of the significance of a background of a common experience of childbearing.

Another aspect of midwifery which has been addressed by this book emerged unsurprisingly in Elaine's chapter on the ex-midwife. In Chapter 13 by Dennis, however, he also addressed the decision of whether to continue as a midwife. This decision is one which will, hopefully, be assisted by the publication of this book.

An aspect of midwifery that may certainly need more attention is one that emerges out of Valerie's writing in Chapter 11 on the global midwife. This is the political nature of what the midwife does or does not do. This aspect of midwifery may have been ignored in favour of a focus on the care of the mother and baby that the midwife provides. It is an aspect, though, that midwives neglect at their peril, especially in view of the debate about midwives' professional status.

An issue still needing to be addressed

Probably because the contributors have been chosen for the high level of their expertise in both midwifery and writing about it, there is one particular issue that has not emerged. This issue is unrelated to the more precise pictures of midwifery that, hopefully, have been addressed by this book. This issue is the widespread, even ubiquitous, ignorance of what midwifery in reality is all about.

It should probably come as no surprise that the public have little understanding of the true nature of midwifery practice. Some older members of the public may retain the romanticised picture of midwifery, which is occasionally advanced in the genre of writing that has become known as 'faction', such as the work of Worth (2008). If a more serious historical picture is sought, more authoritative sources are available, such as Reid (2007). For the vast majority of women in the UK, their experience of midwifery is what happens in the maternity hospital to which they are sent to give birth, or more likely 'deliver'. The public see midwives practising in a highly medicalised setting in which their role is, at best, subservient to that of medical practitioners and, at worst, totally invisible. The invisible midwife has become famous or even notorious, in that midwives' conviction of their supportiveness for women leads them to adopt a low profile. Unfortunately, that profile may become so low as to render the midwife indistinguishable.

The extent to which midwives have collaborated in achieving such invisibility is debatable. Their tendency to wear the same clothing as other health care professionals when working in clinical settings makes them less easily distinguishable. This sorry situation is likely to be aggravated, at least in Scotland, by the imposition of a new 'National Uniform' (NHS Scotland 2008).

The media have made no small contribution to the public uncertainty about what the midwife does. Although the media are now more comfortable using the 'm-word', they find it difficult to detach it from 'nursing'. The problems associated with this form of 'bonding' were outlined in the Introduction.

Having suggested that there may be some who are endowed with a limited perception of what midwifery involves, it may be necessary to contemplate midwives' views of their own profession or occupational group. This contemplation leads to the observation that some midwives' understanding of their own practice may leave more than a little to be desired. This point has been brought home forcibly to me when midwifery colleagues have sought to persuade me that, having become qualified as a nurse before I became a midwife, automatically makes me more of a nurse than a midwife. The falsity of this argument is apparent in the fact that, at that time, there was no alternative but to become a nurse in order to become a midwife. Possibly arising out of this, to me, fallacious argument are the midwives who espouse their close links with medical practitioners. This group has been dubbed 'medwives' by those midwives who are less than sympathetic to this stance. What this scenario has involved is that some midwives have colluded with medical practitioners to convert childbearing from its healthy, physiological, bio-psychosocial experience into a series of technological interventions. Thus, it may be that many UK midwives have, either willingly or under duress, transformed themselves into 'medwives'.

While clearly far from ideal, this title may be appropriate if we consider the origins of the term 'midwife'. It originates from the Old English term meaning 'with woman'. Medwife is obviously not an accurate translation, but it does imply that such practitioners prefer to align themselves with their medical colleagues, rather than to 'be with' the women for whom they provide care. Mavis Kirkham has presented this person's position as an explicit choice, whereby the midwife is required to choose between being either 'with woman' or 'with medic'. Adopting a characteristically and appropriately 'stroppy' stance, Kirkham argues that there is no room for compromise or occupying the middle ground in this matter.

Concluding words

This difficulty in understanding what midwifery is about is clearly not confined to the lay public. It is a challenge that may be shared by a large number of people involved in health care. Many of these people should certainly know better than to be so ill-informed. Where does the reason for this lack of understanding lie? Could it be that midwives' traditional and probably quite appropriate focus on the care that they provide to mothers and their babies has led them to disregard the need to give attention to, what may be termed in media jargon, their 'image'?

It is possible that this book may serve to remedy this deficiency. By demonstrating the reality of what it is that twenty-first century midwives actually do, it is not only the potential midwives and the experienced midwives who will be given food for thought.

References

Department of Health (DH) (1993) *Changing Childbirth*, Report of the Expert Maternity Group, London: HMSO.

NHS Scotland (2008) 'National Uniform'. Available online at www.scotland. gov.uk/Topics/Health/NHS-Scotland/uniform/uniform1/Q/editmode/on/ forceupdate/on (accessed 12 January 2009).

Reid, L. (2007) *Scottish Midwives: Twentieth century voices*, Fife: Black Devon Books.

Worth, J. (2008) *Call The Midwife: A true story of the East End in the 1950s*, London: Phoenix.

Glossary

Amni-hook A disposable instrument used to rupture the membranes (Smyth *et al.* 2007; see also **ARM**).

ARM (artificial rupture of membranes) Also known as an amniotomy. An intervention by midwives and others intended to augment or accelerate labour (Smyth *et al.* 2007).

CTG (cardiotocograph) A record of the foetal heart rate in relation to the mother's contractions. Some CTGs can confuse the mother's and baby's heart rates, which may cause the operator to miss problems with the baby.

Elective A phenomenon that is chosen, but often used to mean a Caesarean that is planned, as opposed to an emergency operation. In this context, the term gives no indication of who makes the plans or the reason for the Caesarean.

Flat A term used to describe a newborn baby suffering from respiratory depression.

HDU (high-dependency unit) The area where care is provided for women with serious health problems.

Keys Usually refers to the keys (among others) of the controlled drugs cupboard. These keys are ordinarily carried by the midwife in administrative charge of the ward or unit, so they may have some symbolic significance. The midwife 'in charge', though, will give the keys to any midwife needing to administer a controlled drug.

ME (myalgic encephalomyelitis) Also known as 'chronic fatigue syndrome', a medical condition of unknown cause, with fever, aching and prolonged tiredness and depression (*OD* 2000).

Multigravida A woman having her second or subsequent baby.

OP (occipito-posterior position) A position of the foetal head in the mother's pelvis that is associated with a long labour.

Paed   Paediatrician.

PPH (post-partum haemorrhage)   Serious bleeding, usually via the vagina, after the birth of a baby.

Synto   Depending on the context: (a) syntocinon – a synthetic form of the naturally occurring posterior pituitary hormone oxytocin, which (among other effects) causes uterine contractions; or (b)syntometrine – a combination of syntocinon and ergometrine, a similar oxytocic substance. Syntometrine is widely used in the active management of the third stage of labour (McDonald and Prendiville 1992).

References

McDonald, S. and Prendiville, W.J. (1992) 'A randomized controlled trial of syntocinon vs syntometrine . . .', *Journal of Perinatal Medicine* 20(1): 97.

Oxford Dictionary (*OD*) (2000) 'Chronic fatigue syndrome', Oxford: Oxford University Press.

Smyth, R.M.D., Alldred, S.K. and Markham, C. (2007) 'Amniotomy for shortening spontaneous labour', *Cochrane Database of Systematic Reviews* 4. Available online at DOI: 10.1002/14651858, Art. No. CD006167.pub2.

Index